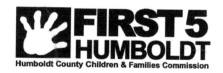

FIRST 5
HUMBOLDT
Humboldt County Children & Families Commission

Boys of Few Words

Boys of Few Words

Raising Our Sons to Communicate
and Connect

. . .

Adam J. Cox, PhD

THE GUILFORD PRESS
New York   London

© 2006 Adam J. Cox
Published by The Guilford Press
A Division of Guilford Publications, Inc.
72 Spring Street, New York, NY 10012
www.guilford.com

The information in this volume is not intended as a substitute for consultation with health care professionals. Each individual's health concerns should be evaluated by a qualified professional.

The individuals and families described in this book, with the exception of the author's own, are composites of the author's clinical work and life experiences. In the interest of confidentiality, names and other identifying information have been changed.

Printed in the United States of America

This book is printed on acid-free paper.

Last digit is print number: 9   8   7   6   5   4   3   2   1

Library of Congress Cataloging-in-Publication Data

Cox, Adam J.
    Boys of few words : raising our sons to communicate and connect / Adam J. Cox.
        p.   cm.
    Includes bibliographical references and index.
    ISBN 1-59385-208-8 (trade paper) — ISBN 1-59385-218-5 (trade cloth)
    1. Boys.   2. Child rearing.   3. Communication in the family.   I. Title.
    HQ775.C68 2006
    649'.132—dc22
                                                          2005014039

For Addison,
whose joy has set my life to song

Contents

■ ■ ■

Part III

How to Make Lasting Differences
■

Acknowledgments

■ ■ ■

T here are many people who contributed to bringing this book to life. The most important contributors, however, are the boys who have inspired its writing. I heartily thank them for what they have taught me about themselves, and also thank their families for entrusting me with their care. The privilege has been mine. I also want to express my appreciation to the many schools that have invited me to be a part of consulting about the challenges of specific boys. The teachers, administrators, and guidance counselors with whom I have worked have been great allies in many ways. Hillside School, in particular, has shown me how creative and dedicated educators can be, and I am very grateful to have been their partner in meeting the social learning needs of children in my community.

Several people, including George Bartlett, Chuck Canfield, and Sue Straeter, were especially helpful in guiding my thoughts about the relationship between families and schools. I thank them for their willingness to share their wisdom and advice.

By way of collaboration, I have met many pediatricians, family doctors, and other health care providers who share a collective passion for improving children's health and emotional well-being. I am appreciative of those who have demonstrated their trust in my ability to be of assistance to their patients and especially thank Dr. John Heid, Dr. Carol Hunter, and their excellent staff for a collegial and productive working relationship.

When I "heard the call" to write this book, Trish Boppert connected me with Margot Maley Hutchison, a literary agent at Waterside Productions, who responded with immediate and unwavering support for what was then little more than a sketchy e-mail. Margot's belief in this project brought me to The Guilford Press, where I have had the good fortune to work with a stellar editorial group including Kitty Moore, Chris Benton, and Sarah Lavender Smith. Their consistent enthusiasm and insight have helped me "take this book to the next level." I can't imagine a better working relationship than I have had with Guilford.

At my office I was ably assisted by Laura Walker, who diligently transcribed the manuscript over the year and a half that it took to complete. I have also benefited from the assistance of Dianne Gehman and Nanette Balliet-Exley, who so thoughtfully managed my clinical practice, allowing me to turn my attention to such things as writing a book. I also want to express my appreciation to the other clinicians in my practice, Daniel Werner, PsyD, Kimberley Katz-Napolitano, MSW, Danielle Goodwin, PsyD, and Meredith Mitstifer, MS, for sharing a commitment to the healthy development of individuals and families, and for conveying their perspectives about many interesting and complex cases over the past several years.

As much as my education and training have informed my thoughts and advice, there is no doubt that much of my thinking stems from the memories of a terrific childhood. I warmly thank my parents, Larry and Gail Cox, for providing me with a foundation that has enabled and motivated me to nurture others. The gifts of my own family are no less substantial. Addison has given me the great pleasure of fatherhood and has enjoyed offering his own insights on boys, although I know he was glad when Daddy's book was finally done!

To my wife, Jacquelyne, I express my deepest thanks. Her love and belief are as important to my life as oxygen, and her countless readings of the manuscript are an unrepayable debt. Our many conversations about parenting, and the creative ideas that followed, are the essence of this book's spirit.

BOYS OF FEW WORDS

Prologue

■ ■ ■

This is a book about the psychology of boys. It has grown out of my clinical work with boys between the age of four and late adolescence over the past decade. I wrote it for parents who want to have a close and loving relationship with their sons and who want to deeply know their minds and hearts. My aim has been to give you a road map to help your son forge healthy relationships, without fear or limitations.

The boys we'll discuss are a diverse group, characterized by communication challenges that threaten to limit their social and emotional development. Most struggle to find the words they need to define their feelings and thoughts and, as a result, miss important opportunities to participate in all that life has to offer. I refer to them as "boys of few words," a reference to the expression "man of few words," so often used to describe someone who expresses himself through actions more easily than language or who may be known for his stoic reserve. The question to consider—at the very heart of this book—is whether this type of social disposition is a viable approach to living a successful life in the twenty-first century. Because this concern is so important, we'll explore how to make meaningful differences in our sons' lives and how we can help them become men capable of being "strong" in multiple ways.

In parenting boys of few words, nurturing their social and communication skills promises the best hope of helping them across the communication divide. This divide represents the gap between stumbling through life with minimally sufficient communication and

building the expressive and social skills required for successful participation in family, school, and community. For parents committed to
understanding their sons, this book examines the relationship between the "male brain" and boys' verbal and social learning challenges. You'll find strategies that can make the difference between
raising a boy who languishes in social detachment or shuts others out
in angry frustration and one who flourishes as a well-rounded, confident, and capable person. The stakes involved are high. Crossing that
gap is about more than improved language skills. It is about better
prospects for being happy, emotionally healthy, and socially competent. Boys who are able to make this critical leap will find themselves
more able to assume positions of leadership in our society, because
they will have the ability to understand, inspire, and relate to others.

My work with boys has not always followed a clear path. Yet I
have learned that if we listen to the quiet voice within us, it will often tell us when we're on track. It may be only as loud as a whisper,
but the message can be so important that it causes us to rethink ourselves, changing the very purpose or calling of our life.

In the 1980s, I was an artist working from a storefront studio in
Hoboken, New Jersey, hoping to discover my destiny in the art galler-
ies and museums of New York City. The studio had a grille that rolled
up to admit sunlight through the front windows and a door that
could be propped open to let in some air. The street was a locus of activity, filled with the raucous sounds of urban life. I lived and worked
in this neighborhood, balancing the risks of invasion with the haz-
ards of isolation. I concluded that as an outsider, a "guest" of the
neighborhood, I ought to keep my door open. In addition to adopting a large black cat, I was visited by the children who lived in the
tenements that lined the block. They were curious and naturally receptive to learning about what an artist does. Before long, they
poked in the cabinets, stuck their fingers in the paints, and asked
questions about the paintings I was making. Having no other pa-
trons, I welcomed their interest by explaining my intention to create
art about how the human mind works. My conversations with these
children seemed to spike their own interest in self-expression, and it
wasn't long before I found myself handing out paper and pastels. I
was amazed at their eagerness to relate and how well they grasped
the idea of art. With some amusement, I noted that my art lessons—
proffered as a peace offering I hoped would keep my studio windows
intact—provided a source of inspiration. Even more important is that

I discovered the rewards of working with children—the deep satisfaction of the creativity required to understand and nurture others.

Ultimately, I found the time spent teaching and helping these kids to be a better fit for my temperament and life's purpose than the solitary habits of an artist. I had no idea about the journey I was about to embark on, and certainly no idea that the seeds of my work as a family psychologist had been planted. Yet I now know that those days were among the defining moments of my life, and I thank those children for helping me see that my education wasn't finished and that my calling was not what I had originally thought.

Having followed the call to work with children, I'm eager to share with you what I've learned about parenting boys. As a father, I continue to learn much from raising my own son, but the guidance I offer here stems from my experience consulting with parents and schools about the complex and unique challenges boys present. My views have been formed by considering children's development from multiple perspectives, having worked in colleges and schools, in an adolescent psychiatric inpatient unit, and as the clinical director of my own group mental health practice, specializing in the social and emotional development of children.

To understand why your son may be a "boy of few words," you have to delve into the psychological realities of boyhood, and this is the goal of the first section of this book. Part I will help you take a closer look at your son's communications skills, especially in connection with his social and emotional development, and use checklists to identify specific areas of concern. I'll explain why boys are much more often affected by communication problems than girls and why we need to do everything possible to help boys reach their full potential to communicate. It's language, after all, that helps boys understand their own feelings and identify with those of others, and these abilities are keys to successful relationships throughout life. Why *don't* they talk as much as we expect them to? Boys often seem intent on doing quite the opposite, limiting their communication to shrugging shoulders or concrete answers, or getting angry when we press for more information. The many interconnected reasons for this are explored in Chapter 3, and as we'll see in Chapter 4, if we don't help them develop an adequate language for emotion and social interaction, they may grow up lacking the empathy and emotional literacy that are absolutely essential to success in our increasingly communication-driven world.

Yet social convention tells us that it's typical for boys to be less socially comfortable than girls, leaving many parents confused about when their sons' reticence is a problem. You'll meet dozens of boys in these chapters who may remind you of your own son or other boys you have known. Their words, and those of their parents, portray the insights and struggles of families and are drawn from the many hours I've spent talking to parents about how to support and nurture their sons' development. I hope they will show you the different faces of boys of few words and give you a new understanding of what's behind the masks boys so often use.

Boys have inherent differences that make communication skills a little harder (but by no means impossible!) to come by than for girls. And they are also subject to social pressures that discourage self-expression. But some boys have additional challenges, which will be discussed in Part II. Is your son so shy that he withdraws from peers and even your family? I will help you understand what may be making him retreat into his shell and how you can draw him out. Does your son express himself mainly through anger? For some boys, anger and aggression are the bricks that build walls of social separation. We'll explore how boys often use anger to assert power or to deny the self-consciousness inherent in growing up in Chapter 6. The third group of boys we will discuss are those affected by learning disabilities and related problems at school. In Chapter 7 we'll consider the important relationship between reading skills and social comprehension and examine how attention deficits shape the quality of boys' social interaction. Many boys of few words, and perhaps your own son, will have traits of more than one of these three groups.

What can you do to help a boy of few words? Raising a socially and emotionally competent son requires dedicated attention, but there's so much you can do to help a boy with a problem overcome it or to help a less impaired boy reach his full potential for social communication. Part III offers ten principles to guide the child-centered family, and a thorough list of practical suggestions for addressing whatever concerns you have about your son's communication abilities. You'll find advice for boys of all ages, clearly illustrating what can be done to help your son at home and school. Because teachers can be so helpful in fostering your son's self-awareness and social communication skills, and because school is the center of your son's universe for much of his childhood, we will talk about how you can work strategically with schools on your son's behalf. Finally, we'll consider situations in which your son might benefit from professional help. If you wonder whether professional intervention is in the best interest of your son, you'll find guidance in answering that question, details about the different types of help available, and what will be involved in getting an evaluation in Chapter 11. I hope that these chapters will serve as a resource to which you return many times.

My guess is that you are reading this book because you're concerned about an important boy in your life. Motivated by your love and assisted by your intuition, you can use the tools in this book to help him shine. As we explore how to build the deep, reciprocal relationships that arc life's reward, remember to listen to the quiet voice within you. The experiences of your own life, for better or worse, the experiments, accidents, detours, and surprises that make up *your* personal life story will inform and guide you. No matter what path you have taken, or what has brought you to this place, your interest and care are evident. From here, we can find a way to reach out to the boy who concerns you now.

This path we travel together.

Part I

The Communication Divide

...

ONE

Is Your Son a Boy of Few Words?

■ ■ ■

Five-year-old Jeremy is a small, busy boy with dark hair and a mischievous expression. He's very interested in superheroes and race car drivers. Despite his energy and enthusiasm, he's struggling to adjust to kindergarten. Jeremy's teacher has trouble getting his attention, and he resists joining group activities. Within his first month of school, he pushed one of the other children three times. When his teacher asked him why, he would only repeat, defiantly, "It's not my fault." When his parents made similar inquiries, he "put on his storm face," as his mother calls it, and refused to answer. His parents acknowledge that little things seem to "set him off" and worry that aggression is the primary way Jeremy expresses himself. They wonder if he'll outgrow it or if there's something else they can do—so far, attempts at discipline like time-out only seem to undermine any willingness he has to cooperate or communicate with them.

Aaron is a thin, serious eight-year-old with extraordinary intellectual gifts. Because he reads science fiction voraciously and has a good vocabulary for things related to astronomy or the parts of a "cyborg," his father calls him "the little professor." Despite his strengths, he often seems lost in his own world. His parents wonder if he notices other people and if they notice him. Aaron rarely talks to peers and complains that no one likes him. He looks puzzled when asked to explain the difference between sadness and anger. "He's like the 'invisible' boy. He'll share his thoughts, but not his heart," explained his mother. "When I talk to him about making friends at school or ask him how he's feeling, he immediately changes the subject. The only conversations we have are about facts— what causes a volcano to erupt, how you predict a hurricane, and so forth. I'm proud that he knows about those things, but he doesn't pick up on what other people are interested in. Shouldn't he want more friends?"

Morgan, a tall, heavy-set eleven-year-old, is passionate about fantasy computer games, especially when he can play with someone else. However, his parents complain that other kids don't want to come to the house because Morgan gets so caught up in the game he starts "giving orders," insisting that his peers play the games as he says. When the other kids resist or get bored, Morgan becomes unreasonably frustrated.

Sometimes he acts out, blurring the distinction between the characters in game scenarios and his companions. His mother quietly admits that at times even she feels a little afraid of Morgan. "I think he gets too carried away with the games. He's old enough to realize that a game's just a game and that people matter more, but honestly, if we took away his computer, I'm not sure how he'd react."

Fourteen-year-old Zachary avoids family interaction. He feels excessively self-conscious when asked about his day or anything remotely personal. When his parents try to discuss their concerns with him, he just shrugs and says, "I don't know. Nothing is wrong. Just leave me alone." Zachary is obsessed with building remote control cars and spends hours working on them. Despite his father's hope that this hobby would help their relationship, Zachary works mostly in silence, speaking only when he wants help and only about the cars. "When he's not working on the cars, he lives in his room," complains his mother. "When I ask, 'What are you up to?' he grunts. When I ask, 'What did you do in school?' he says, 'Nothing.' Sometimes it feels like we're strangers to him. I don't know how this happened."

These are just a few examples of how the communication difficulties of boys become manifest in their daily lives. You may see them take shape as withdrawal, indifference, anger, depression, a combination of these traits, or something that looks entirely different to you. Your parental instincts suggest something might be wrong—but what? All you can really be sure of is that your son's communication has become infrequent or unexpectedly distant for someone you feel so close to.

How many times have you wondered what's going on in your son's mind or felt confused or frustrated by his apparent inability to express himself? Maybe you've felt the sting of his disinterest in relating to you. Even within the most loving parent–child relationship, connecting with boys can be a difficult, sometimes thankless task. Yet helping your son across the communication divide is an expression of your commitment to care for his social development and is one of the most enduring gifts you will ever give him.

Your concern demonstrates that you've already started to make that commitment. One of my principal goals is to offer specific interventions—ways to communicate with your son, draw out his self-expression, and create a nurturing family atmosphere—that you can use to help your son cross the communication divide. But your efforts to apply them will be most successful if they are supported by an understanding of why the task is so important and what your son is up against.

Why It's So Important to Nurture Communication in Boys

Communication skills help boys move beyond using speech for merely functional requests ("Can I watch TV?") or information retrieval ("Can we buy it?"). Our sons cross the communication divide when they begin using communication for self-definition ("I feel . . . I believe . . . I hope . . . I am . . . "). Learning to use expressive communication helps clear a path to a life full of mutually satisfying relationships and paves the way for greater personal and professional opportunities in adulthood. These are the stakes when it comes to talking about the *social communication* skills of boys.

Success in School and at Work Depends More Than Ever on Communication

Although boys today may have better vocabularies and more varied social opportunities than males of generations ago, *the communication difficulties of boys are more noticeable than ever.* This is because the societal demand to communicate and relate effectively is growing progressively stronger—faster than the pace at which the social communication skills of boys are developing. This discrepancy only highlights the communication divide, the growing gap between many boys' current social and communication skills and the level of ability required for full participation in social and vocational life in the twenty-first century.

The visibility of socially disconnected boys has grown steadily over the last hundred years because there are far fewer nonverbal, asocial lifestyle and vocational options. Socially challenged males are, unfortunately, destined to stick out or seem out of place if we don't act to reverse this trend. We are already beginning to see how the communication divide has contributed to characterizing the class structures of our time. In this century, your son is statistically unlikely to work the land or be a lonesome cowboy. Success in school, which rests squarely on the presumption that language is the basis of learning, is an expectation that society and most parents insist on. Few vocational options remain that don't rely heavily on social perception and communication. In fact, the business community has thoroughly embraced the concept of "emotional intelligence" (EQ)—

a new emphasis on the value of emotional awareness that promotes personal health and successful relationships. The business world has learned that it literally cannot afford to ignore the contribution these skills make to organizational life. We live in increasingly complex, interactive, and crowded systems. Whether at home or school, boys are challenged to express what they think and feel, especially if they want their thoughts and feelings to count for something—if they want to be heard.

> ■ ■ ■
>
> As an adult, your son is more likely to negotiate a contract than a mountain pass, to work on the phone than work on the land. Will he be ready?

As a society, are we prepared to gamble that the growth of "technical jobs" and electronic communication will eliminate the need to manage basic social hurdles such as family life, friendship, courtship, and parenthood? The foundation for managing those hurdles is the capacity to use language as a tool for personal expression and social connection. And even the technological jobs that seem to insulate workers from face-to-face contact require skillful communication. How often have you seen an office crisis sparked by an ill-considered, cryptic, or poorly written e-mail?

In part, the communication challenges of boys have become more visible as the result of dramatic social changes in how people interact. In your son's twenty-first-century education, career, and relationships, he'll be expected to participate in highly social networks. His success will hinge on how well he can access and join those networks. And we cannot afford to wait until our sons are adults to get concerned about this reality. The demand to communicate and engage socially is happening right now, this very day, whether your son has just started preschool or is graduating from college.

Authentic Self-Expression Is Limited by the Erosion of Language

In some ways, the difficulty of becoming an effective social communicator stems from the gradual erosion of language, as it is subject to increasing levels of fragmentation. Sentence syntax (organizational flow) has been reinvented by electronic/media culture—not surprisingly, the preferred "input" source for many boys. Although the creativity reshaping how we use language may be extraordinary, it has led to virtual chaos. Parents may get upset when their sons talk "gangsta," "techno," or "jock," but those language influences ring loudly in your son's mind because they've become highly commercialized and appeal strongly to the emotions and self-absorption of youth culture. Complete sentences have arguably become an endangered species. The glib, cocky nature of commercial communication has contributed to boys' hesitation to communicate and express themselves more authentically. Their need to use authentic communication is no less, but the supply of safe opportunities to do so has diminished. Ironically, the Internet has become one of the few places that males, boys included, are comfortable being vulnerable. Unfortunately, this type of conditioning is counterproductive to healthy social development, and rationalizing that "talking on the Internet is better than nothing" doesn't really help.

Most Boys Don't Appreciate What They're Missing

Here's the catch. Boys are unlikely to recognize the extraordinary life advantages good communication skills confer—at least while they are still children. Most boys would probably smirk at the idea that communication skills are a "gift," even if you could get their attention long enough for them to consider the offering. For important reasons, boys are generally not well suited to appreciate the benefits of social communication.

For one thing, they are so often on the move, physically and psychologically. When their eyes rarely meet ours, it can lead us to wonder, "Did he hear me?"; "Am I getting through?"; "What does he think about what I'm saying?"; "When did he learn to act like this, and from whom?"

Another reason is that boys are clearly different from girls. I don't mean "worse" or "better" in any way. But my clinical experience, reinforced by ample investigation and research data on the subject, has shown that there are definite differences in the routes by which males arrive at their communication skills. Boys' brains work differently in some significant ways, and the thoughts and concerns that fill their minds are distinctly male. Although sometimes these differences can appear subtle, they can dramatically impact the ways that boys behave, especially when it comes to communication. (And yes, communication *is* a behavior.)

Sometimes we *hear* the differences between boys and girls before we *see* them. Adrienne, the mother of two boys and two girls, puts it this way: "The girls are always tuned in to what's happening with me, with each other, with the whole family. They're always talkative and very social. The boys storm in, clear out the snacks, and hit the video games. Major parts of family life bypass them—they're oblivious! If I want to get one of the boys' attention or ask him a question, sometimes I have to literally stand in front of him, repeat his name, and wave my arms. Even then, the response I get is barely more than 'Huh?' or 'I don't know.' It's not that they're unintelligent, but sometimes it's like talking to a wall. If my girls didn't respond so differently, I'd think it was me."

Then there's the world we live in. In the 1980s, as computers became a way of daily life for the average person, and throughout the 1990s as Internet access became commonplace in family households, we frequently heard about the Information Age, a time when the efficient exchange of information would be of paramount importance. It is not a coincidence that both the design and enthusiasm for such a scenario came largely from males. This is because *for many males, the content of communication is far more important than its form*. In fact, this is one of the ways in which males and females tend to differ. For many, although not all, females communication is a fundamental part of life that is intrinsically interesting and rewarding. In contrast, males often perceive communication as far more functional. And at the extreme end, for some men, communication is not a relational or creative process at all but a utilitarian act aimed at getting something they need or want—information. Although the efficient exchange of information through e-mail, instant messaging, or other innovations has its advantages, we should be concerned about a reciprocal downshift in our expressive capabilities. Yet in working with boys, I've noticed how frequently their communication patterns mimic the sparse functionality of mechanical communication. As a consequence, the ability to reflect on their emotions, the capacity to hold opposing thoughts in mind simultaneously, and the social instincts that guide our relationships truly "don't compute."

When boys adopt this type of utilitarian approach to communication, they are shortchanged. This is why it's so important that we recognize and adapt to the complexities of a boy's communication challenges before his possibilities have become unnecessarily limited. We must accept that we live in a world increasingly bound by the need to communicate and relate to others. Through communication we navigate the maze of experiences and relationships that make up

■ ■ ■

It's easy—especially for a mother or a sister—to view a boy as uncaring or rude when his conversation seems terse or perfunctory: "Give me the milk." "Aunt Ellen's spaghetti tastes weird—what does she put in it?" "Hurry up, I'm tired of playing this game." "Don't say stupid things when my friends come over, okay?" But some boys understand communication as a purely functional exercise, aimed at getting or providing necessary information. Appreciating that your son is probably not aware of how his words are received can help you turn such interactions into a teaching opportunity about the impact of his communication. Does he know that the way he says something is as important as what he might say?

a life—at home, school, and, eventually, work. Communication helps us define and know our emotional selves, making us more well rounded, better prepared to fully participate in the world.

Unfortunately, boys' relatively limited life experience does not give them access to such privileged information. As concerned parents, we should understand the value of communication as an element of self-development that enriches life and contributes to better psychological adjustment. Even buoyed by our convictions about the value of good communication skills, teaching them can be a daunting challenge. In part, this is because boys are often reluctant to work at things that don't come easily, particularly when they don't naturally sense how communication and relationships are so deeply intertwined. Social communication skills begin with a willingness to be expressive and to share a part of oneself with others. Self-expression invariably requires some degree of vulnerability, and as we will see, this is a fearful prospect for many boys.

The Signs of Problems Are Too Easy to Miss

Whether at home or at school, boys are rarely expected to be as verbal as girls. Because boys often seem to have an innate preference for expressing themselves through action versus language, it can be easy to miss or ignore signs of expressive language problems. Although most of us would likely agree that it is good for boys to communicate, social and expressive deficits may be overlooked in families where boys are more celebrated for their physical development, athletic ability, or skills in mastering more technical tasks. In our culture, the image of a happy little boy is one of a kid running around being busy, playing, jumping, running, throwing things, perhaps getting into a little mischief. If this is your little boy, he may not slow down long enough for you to notice if his expressive abilities are delayed. Yet as such boys mature, language deficits nobody noticed may "take root" and become part of their psychological makeup. Expressive problems lead to the emergence of social and emotional difficulties: boys have impoverished vocabularies for emotions and cannot "put their finger on" how they are feeling. Consequently, they struggle to manage or control difficult feelings and may be at a serious loss to read the emotions of others. In turn, this type of emotional illiteracy limits a boy's capacity to successfully initiate or sustain relationships. Incredibly, before many boys have even finished elementary school, they have silently concluded that they are socially incompetent. And as is so often true for boys, when they decide they are not good at something, they become disinterested. This briefly described sequence of events is a glimpse of how communication difficulties lead boys to project an attitude of social indifference. When we see the mask of indifference emerge, we can reasonably assume it's being used to hide a lack of confidence and declining self-esteem, at least with respect to social communication.

Few boys want to show that they're affected by communication challenges, yet despite their stone-faced expressions and shoulder shrugging, the hurt and frustration are palpable. Think about how exasperating it is to have as much emotion as anybody else, without adequate ability to vent or verbally explore that emotion. If you look and listen closely, you'll recognize that the hard, stoic front many boys put on is camouflage for a world of unexpressed feeling. Now think about how often you've seen boys (as well as men) at play, dressed in camouflage garb! Boys are infatuated with how to go undetected and how that skill can be an element of power or advantage. Whether by clothing or constricted body language, boys explore the application of camouflage in their play and in managing relationships where they feel vulnerable.

Self-constructed defenses are not the only way social communication deficits of boys are shielded from view. Behavioral problems such as defiance, social anxiety, attention-deficit/hyperactivity disorder (ADHD), and learning disabilities—all of which disproportionately affect males—also mask expressive and receptive communication problems. Untangling the reciprocal relationship of behavioral and learning problems with communication deficits is a classic "chicken or egg" question that can perplex the best of parents and professionals alike.

I believe we need to detect communication problems much earlier in boys' lives and act to prevent the kind of social standoff that results from these problems as boys get older. As we'll see, the self-consciousness associated with poor social skills becomes amplified in adolescence, as boys become more focused on how they compare to peers. Having to get through to adolescent boys who have withdrawn into isolation from fear or repeated frustration makes a parent's job much harder.

What Your Son Is Up Against: Key Neuropsychological Differences between Boys and Girls

Research over the last few decades has shown that neuropsychology—the interaction of the brain and a person's psychology—is an area of great relevance to the way boys perceive and relate to their social environment. Therefore, learning some basics about neuropsychology will help you understand the uniqueness of boys and how to coach them across the communication divide. Keep in mind, however, that biology is not destiny; the fact that there are brain differences between boys and girls does not give us license to ignore boys' communication and resign ourselves to "boys being boys." This perspective defeats the very purpose of exploring this information. There is not a person alive who does not have some type of behavioral liability due to personality, development, or genetics. The real difference between us is how well we manage those liabilities. Where children are concerned, a good deal of the management lies in the choices parents make about how to respond to their children's needs.

Boys Beware: Greater Risk of Neurological Disorders

One of the first things to know about the liabilities of boys is that they are much more vulnerable than girls (about 4–5:1) to a wide range of neurological disorders, including learning disabilities, ADHD, autism, and a host of variants of these syndromes. Interesting to note is that *all of these syndromes typically encompass some type of*

■ ■ ■

The quality of a boy's communication can help you understand his psychological and emotional reality. Before assuming poor communication stems from a lack of effort, consider whether it reflects some kind of neurological difference that requires attention.

problem with communication. Again and again, we'll see that the quality of a boy's communication is a revealing window into his psychological, social, and emotional well-being.

Several prominent theories attempt to explain why males seem to be so much more vulnerable to neurodevelopmental problems, including gender differences in the anatomy of the brain, the role of testosterone in prenatal development, qualitative differences in how boys and girls are socialized and taught, and the infatuation that boys have with electronic media and games, typically beginning in early childhood. All of these theories seem to hold at least a grain of truth, although no single explanation has been "certified" as the definitive answer. Scientists have established strong genetic links for some of the syndromes I have noted, yet these issues continue to be debated intensely. Luckily, some of the best epidemiologists in the world are working on solving this clinical puzzle and will undoubtedly contribute to our understanding of boys' vulnerability to these problems in the years to come. In other parts of this book, Chapter 7 in particular, I'll help you figure out whether one of these neurodevelopmental problems could be playing a role in your son's communication difficulties.

Like most psychological phenomena, communication problems have multiple causes and effects. This stems in part from the fact that the development of a child's brain is extraordinarily intricate and subtle. Just as each child's life is socially unique, shaped by variables like family life, class issues, or cultural identity, neurodevelopment is also unique, shaped by the quality of a child's learning opportunities and the idiosyncrasies of biology.

■ ■ ■

Scientists are working hard to understand the causes of the neurodevelopmental differences of boys. But even when we have more answers, we will need to accept that gender-based brain differences are not likely to change soon and that boys will require a helping hand when it comes to developing the communication skills they need.

Is Your Son Well "Connected"?

Although the brain has many parts, some with relatively well-defined functions, each part relies to some degree on all the others through an elaborate communication network of brain cells called *neurons*. This makes all the different areas and systems of the brain highly interdependent, in the same way that the sound of a symphony depends on all the different instruments and the musicians who play them. Communication is one example of a behavior that depends on a complex combination of activities in the brain. In fact, it's impossible to overstate how important it is to becoming an effective communicator that a boy's perceptual skills (how his senses detect new information) and processing skills (how he organizes and comprehends that information) be fully integrated. For example, if the parts of his brain that handle perception are compromised or underdeveloped, he may not be able to translate or process information very well. When an instrument is removed from the arrangement of a musical score, the sound and feeling will be noticeably different too.

When it comes to receiving communication, our ability to detect visual cues can be just as important as what we hear. Consider how people's body language, for example, their expression or hand movements, might help you understand their feelings or what they're trying to say. In fact, our brains can process large amounts of visual information much more efficiently than we can process a large amount of auditory information. For example, suppose you go into a job interview. Before the interviewer says anything, in a few seconds you've noted that he's looking at you skeptically, leaning back in his chair, has a precise haircut, blue eyes, and is a sharp dresser. Now think about how hard it is to listen to even just two things at the same time. You probably get a little irritated if you're trying to pay attention to someone and somebody else starts talking to you at the same time. This is because we process auditory information in a more linear, sequential manner than we do visual information. Perhaps one of the reasons we frequently hear that "most communication is nonverbal" is that, generally speaking, our brains are more efficient at processing larger quantities of nonverbal information. My point is that becoming an effective social communicator requires boys to make important connections between what they hear *and* what they see. It is in combining these two basic pathways of perception that a person has the best chance of understanding and staying connected to others. If we are to have a meaningful impact on our sons' communication, we will have to teach them to notice and interpret the visual cues that enrich social interaction.

Can You Hear Me Now?

In general, girls are better at processing language than boys. This fact alone goes a long way toward explaining why girls overall have better communication skills than boys. In a sense, girls hear language more deeply, using more of their brain to process and understand language than do boys. This expanded processing capability adds up to additional social perception and the versatility to use that knowledge in social communication.

■ ■ ■

When girls hear language, they're better able to make inferences that shape the meaning of what was said. On the morning Vivian was getting married, her sister Theresa hugged her, smiled, and said, "Oh, I'm going to cry." Vivian immediately understood that Theresa was expressing joy, but their brother asked, "What's wrong with Theresa?" In such situations, males of all ages have a tendency to think in more literal terms, sometimes undermining their ability to grasp the full meaning of a person's communication.

The auditory processing advantages of girls also carry over into the classroom, where girls generally develop better vocabularies and learn to read earlier than boys. A general rule of human nature is that when you have a particular talent, you tend to use it. By extension, most girls learn to enjoy the expressive capabilities of language because they are very effective at using them. Communication simply comes more easily for most girls.

Although the auditory processing skills of girls generally surpass those of boys, we should recognize that some boys are good auditory learners. You'll know who these boys are, because you can tell they rely on listening skills as a primary learning pathway. For example, if you want to teach these boys how to introduce themselves, they'll learn that skill best by listening to what you say and rehearsing the words and phrases themselves. By contrast, boys who are visual learners will be more focused on watching how to introduce themselves and committing to memory a sequence of images related to introductions.

Although visually oriented boys may face some auditory learning challenges, they are not usually the boys who struggle with listening skills the most. That distinction belongs to boys who tend to rely on kinesthetics (movement and touch) to process and learn new information. These boys love to be active, exploring and learning about their environment through physical contact and the movement of their bodies through space. You may have met boys who want to handle and touch everything—learning through their fingertips—or who immediately check out or map a new place by investigating its perimeter. Boys with this learning orientation typically love the outdoors and are in bliss when given a new territory to explore. (They are also the boys most likely to push the boundaries of that territory, such as by riding their bikes past points you have designated.)

Because words are a less relevant source of information input for kinesthetically oriented boys, you can imagine what happens when these kids go to school. Nearly everything is auditory or visual, and there are generally strict rules about what can be touched, handled, or climbed on. As a consequence, these boys often feel like fish out of water. Verbal processing is secondary for many of these boys, and as a result, they often present a disinterested face to the process of learning. This unfortunate situation results in all types of misdiagnoses. For example, if verbal learning feels unnatural to a boy, it's highly likely that he'll have difficulty sustaining attention, and as a result, will appear distracted to a teacher. A similar phenomenon can occur

■ ■ ■

Do you know a boy who needs to handle everything, is uncomfortable with direct eye contact, likes to spread out and make himself very comfortable on furniture, explores a new space by walking or running around it, or needs to show his anger through physical contact rather than words? Could he be a kinesthetic learner who will learn better by doing than watching or listening? Kinesthetic boys are often less inclined toward verbal communication, but they still have important things to say. Parents will do better at inviting their verbal participation when using words that resonate for these boys. Rather than saying, "Do you *see* what I mean?" or "Can you *hear* my point?" try, "What would *feel like a good fit* to you?" or "Your observation really *hit the mark.*"

at home, as boys appear oblivious to the comments of parents or siblings. It's not that being a kinesthetic learner gets a boy off the hook when it comes to succeeding as a communicator. The demands of our society make that an unacceptable option. Still, we cannot be truly helpful to these boys unless we acknowledge their special challenges and incorporate that understanding into our approach to helping.

Interestingly, girls and boys also seem to differ with respect to what *kinds* of sounds they hear most clearly. In their fascinating book, *Brain Sex,* Anne Moir and David Jessel note that while girls are better at imitating the sounds of human speech, boys excel when it comes to replicating machine and animal sounds. This discrepancy seems to speak to each gender's evolutionary path, with males and females having become especially attuned to sounds that dominated their respective daily activities and responsibilities. For males, these activities have often centered on hunting, tool making, and building. Elements of these activities are clearly evident in the play of boys today. I believe many parents of boys would agree that a notable component of boys' play is their fascination with how things work, a trait that can be observed in boys from a very young age.

At least one notable researcher has theorized that boys are fascinated with how things work because they are "systematizers." In his book *The Essential Difference,* Dr. Simon Baron-Cohen, a psychologist and leading autism researcher, suggests that males and females can be broadly categorized as "systematizers" and "empathizers," respectively. In his thought-provoking book he explores how these tendencies explain many of the social differences we see between males and females, particularly why males are less attuned to interpersonal exchange. For Baron-Cohen, these differences also explain why autism is so much more prevalent among males, suggesting that autism can be understood as an extreme form of maleness! Although this theory requires further investigation, my personal experience has shown me that while girls as young as seven can engage in short-duration, talk-based therapy, boys of the same age will predictably require some type of game or activity as a background to talking in order for them to be comfortable.

Bridging the Gap

It turns out that girls learn language skills more easily than boys in part because girls are uniquely able to use a much larger part of the brain to process language. While brain imaging studies have shown that boys process language almost exclusively with their left hemisphere, girls can more effectively engage both hemispheres in language processing. In addition, they can share information between hemispheres by virtue of a part of the brain called the *corpus callosum*. This structure is essentially a bundle of fibers that spans the two hemispheres, acting like a bridge over which information can be transferred between the left and right hemisphere. Although recent research shows that the differences may not be as great as was once thought, the corpus callosum is consistently larger (more bulbous) in girls than in boys, facilitating more efficient exchange of information between the hemispheres—just as a wider bridge moves traffic from one side to the other more quickly. The net result is that language processing in boys is more likely to be limited to the processing capabilities of the left hemisphere, while girls are generally better able to apply right-hemisphere capabilities to their symphony of communication skills.

What kind of advantage does this confer on girls? The left hemisphere of the brain is where we process spoken and written language. It is also the part of the brain primarily responsible for reasoning, problem solving, and the skills we need to understand most topics in science and math. In contrast, the right hemisphere has more to do with our creativity, insight, and sensitivity to nonverbal information—in essence, the right hemisphere fuels our social intuition. These right-hemisphere perceptual capabilities are more readily available to girls, helping them to complement the left hemisphere's functional processing of language with the insight and social comprehension ability of the right hemisphere.

This is not to say that boys can't or don't have good right-hemisphere skills. The ability to map out space, largely a right-hemisphere skill, is something that males excel in, for example. Still, if, as research continues to suggest, boys use less of their brains in processing language, they are at a decided disadvantage when it comes to learning and using communication skills. And another disadvantage of boys related to right-versus-left hemisphere processing is that they tend to take a left-hemisphere (systematizing) approach to problem solving. While an orientation toward systematic thinking may help males focus on solutions in a goal-directed manner, it also tends to inhibit awareness of the more subtle information that enriches social perception and communication. This situation probably

■ ■ ■

In their rush to solve a problem, boys often overemphasize technicalities and underemphasize social considerations. A student in Galen's class complained that nobody ever sat next to her. Galen suggested to his teacher that she devise a rotating seating chart so this student would eventually sit next to every student on at least one class day. Galen didn't get the point that the student was concerned that nobody seemed to want to sit next to her and that her feelings had been hurt. Do you know boys like Galen who are so anxious for solutions that they miss important messages?

doesn't surprise many females—who may have had to cope with this conundrum for decades.

"You Never Told Me That!"

With respect to memory, girls are better able than boys to re-tain random information in short-term memory, while boys excel at retaining information of personal importance. For example, the dates of birthdays, where something was left, an offhand comment, even what to pick up at the store, are often remembered more easily by females. In general, I believe this helps to explain the apparent self-absorption of many males throughout life. Forgive us, but we males are simply more apt to be interested in and remember things that accentuate what we perceive to be our strengths. Perhaps this ex-

■ ■ ■

As compared with girls, most boys have brain differences that can make learning social communication skills more difficult. These factors include:

- A smaller, less efficient corpus callosum, the bridge that transfers information between our two brain hemispheres
- More challenges with auditory processing skills
- More difficulty retaining random information in short-term memory (an especially important difference when we come to our discussion of ADHD in Chapter 7.)

Remember, these are general tendencies. We should measure our success with boys with respect to how well they fulfill their individual potentials.

plains why boys are so much better at remembering how to win at playing a video game than they are at remembering chores after school, the importance of waving to an elderly neighbor, or getting their homework into a backpack.

Too Many Disadvantages to Overcome?

If you're wondering how your son will have half a chance to become a good communicator with so many potential neuropsychological obstacles to overcome, I ask you to remember two things:

First, we should measure our success with boys with respect to how well each fulfills his individual potential. Don't be too quick to apply the broad statistical tendencies of an entire gender to an individual as unique as your son! There is enough variation among males to produce brilliant orators, writers, and social communicators.

Second, I have yet to meet a boy whose communication skills could not be improved through a steadfast commitment on the part of his parents to make a difference in his social development. This is the contribution that parents can make, and it has enduring value, as successive generations inherit the love, patience, and time you invest in your son.

A Family Perspective

An important message of this book is that the communication problems of boys are very much a family affair. To illustrate the extent to which boys and their families can be affected by communication and social development challenges, let me tell you about a family that came to see me for help with their son. In many respects, this family is like many others I've worked with. I hardly think you could distinguish this boy from his peers, at least in some situations. Yet small problems have a way of becoming bigger problems without adequate attention and intervention.

Jared

Eight-year-old Jared lived with his parents and younger brother, Payne. Jared was fortunate to have loving parents who had worked hard to shape a child-centered family. Family life had flowed along fairly comfortably until Jared started kindergarten. To his parents' surprise, his progress reports were interspersed with occasional negative comments about his "verbal expression" and "friendship skills." Jared's parents thought little of it, assuming that he was just getting used to being in school and that the problems would work themselves out. Although similar reports persisted into first grade, Jared's parents were still not inclined to consider the comments too seriously.

Yet the reports continued, and by second grade Jared was "disruptive to other students," according to a terse note from his teacher. Making matters worse, Jared's problems in school resulted in a great deal of tension between his parents. They disagreed about how to respond to Jared's difficulties. His mother had begun to see related problems at home and felt he needed to be disciplined more strongly or perhaps get counseling: "I can deal with him on days when he's outside running around, but if he's in the house and has to follow some basic rules, it's just chaos." Jared's father felt that Jared was "just being a boy" and that "people should leave him alone." He could recall acting in similar ways when he was Jared's age and didn't understand what all the concern was about. "If Jared is having a problem, the school should deal with it; that's what they get paid for." Jared's mother frowned and shook her head as she heard her husband state his position.

While Jared's parents were trying to come to an agreement about how to handle him, his teacher had requested that he be evaluated by a school psychologist. In addition to noting Jared's problems with expressive language, the school psychologist believed that Jared might have ADHD. When the evaluation results came home, things really got heated up between Jared's parents. Once again, Jared's mother felt validated by the school's suggestions, while his father only grew angrier. "He's an energetic kid—what's wrong with that?" he said.

Parental disagreement about Jared developed into significant marital tension, because Jared's mother saw many of the traits that frustrated her most about her husband in her son as well. When Jared shrugged his shoulders and limited his communication to an occasional "Huh" or "I don't know," his mother would roll her eyes and think, "A total chip off the old block." She was angry with her husband because she felt that he was minimizing her legitimate concerns and she was being overwhelmed by the challenges of helping Jared with his communication skills and behavioral challenges. Before one session, she asked to speak to me privately and complained,

"He's just like his father. I know I sound annoying, but I have to remind both of them over and over to do basic things. I want to help Jared with his school problems, but he'll never talk about it. I'm at the point where I don't want to take him around with me because he's so hard to deal with. I try not to judge him, but it's embarrassing when your child is clueless about what's going on around him, not to mention me." His mother had some very good questions for me: How do you parent a child who cannot focus on you long enough to receive instruction, encouragement, or consequences? And what do you do if this is compounded by the child's inability to express what he is feeling? Although Jared's father still felt that his wife was too quick to accept the judgment of the school, even he admitted that Jared "was a handful."

Jared's parents had brought up a point that arises frequently when families are faced with behavioral challenges in children. Parents often get a lot of advice from well-meaning and critical observers. Because many of us feel that our children are a reflection of ourselves, it can be painful, embarrassing, and lead to a lot of self-doubt when our children behave in less than satisfactory ways. The urgency of some situations can make it difficult to determine if our decisions are based on the best interests of the child or a reaction to the extreme stress of the situation. Jared's father was very sensitive to this issue, fearing that people might be overreacting to Jared's behavior. He wanted to make sure that any decisions made were not reactive, but in his son's best interest. Jared's mother, who as the primary caregiver was "in the trenches" with Jared each day, was concerned that Jared receive the support and treatment she felt he needed.

When children don't appear to be following a normal developmental pattern in communication or behavior, parents want to know if their concerns are warranted. For many, it's a great relief to hear that the best of parents would be overwhelmed by the challenges their child presents. There are some important reasons for this. First, guilt is a perennial parental favorite. When our child seems to lack development or behave in ways we're worried about, we tend to blame ourselves (though sometimes we shift that blame to a spouse or other caretaker). Second, we may find it hard to "benchmark," or compare, our son's behavior with that of other children. You may not have raised other boys or been around boys much in your life. One parent told me, "I thought it was me, but my own mother raised my brothers, and even she says, 'He's a nice boy, but I can't tell if he's listening or understands what I say to him. Does he talk to you?' It was amazing to hear some-one recognize what I deal with every day of my life."

When Jared's parents decided to seek outside help, it was be-cause his teacher was pushing hard for some type of intervention. She recognized that Jared was probably hurting inside, but she had a whole classroom of students to be accountable to. During my evalua-tion of Jared, we looked at how his challenges were impacting the whole family. Along with the marital issues, Jared's mother noted how much easier it was for her to be close to Payne, his younger brother. Despite his being several years younger, Payne's communica-tion skills were more advanced in some important ways. As we talked, Jared's mother realized that because Payne was easier to deal with, their relationship was warmer. "If you smile at him, he beams back. It's unconscious, but I think I smile at him a lot more." Payne's receptivity to communication resulted in his mother's initiating more casual conversation, making more jokes, and generally giving more approval for the things Payne did. More than once she thought to herself, "Jared is like his dad, and his brother is more like me."

This family dynamic probably contributed to the intense sibling rivalry between Payne and Jared. When Payne was younger, he tended to idolize his older brother and Jared enjoyed being the men-tor, the "big boy" who could show his brother how to do things. As Payne matured, however, he noticed that Jared was often in some conflict with his mother and began to take on the role of "the good boy." He also used his superior verbal skills to taunt and tease Jared, who, unable to retaliate verbally, sometimes reacted physically in an-ger. This cycle intensified their mother's frustration.

Jared's parents decided they needed to apply some immediate at-tention to family communication dynamics, which were negatively influencing the course of their family life. It was also clear that Jared needed some individual support to help him understand what he could do to meet expectations and start feeling better about himself in school. To replace his outbursts of rage, we worked on developing an emotional vocabulary (anchored by pictures, because he was a visual learner) to help him discern what he was feeling and develop strategies for coping with those feelings. Jared needed to find effec-tive ways to acknowledge his emotional life.

With boys as young as Jared, play is almost always the focal point for intervention, whether it is in therapy or at home. Play pro-vides virtually unlimited opportunity to explore ideas and feelings and also facilitates the development of new skills like learning to follow rules, social awareness, and communication. Jared's parents and I talked about how we could model communication skills through play. The hours we all have spent interacting with Jared have taught us to be patient and to be attentive to subtle signs of growth in his social and expressive development.

Like many boys of few words, Jared is exceptionally sensitive to feeling inadequate about his expressive capabilities. We've had to work hard at reinforcing his mastery of other skills so that he perceives us as believing in him, even admiring him in some ways. Fortunately, Jared's strengths with puzzles and motor coordination have provided opportunities to give him the type of supportive feedback he craves. We found that relaxing our expectations for Jared, while also expressing our appreciation of his natural talents, urged him to respond by trying to surprise us with a range of social and communication accomplishments he suspected would please—and he was right.

Families mitigate communication and social challenges when they accept their existence and their potential consequences. Seeing your son with open and honest eyes is a basic requirement for positive change. In Jared's case, his parents' honest concern and effort made a tremendous difference. Even their differing perspectives about the approach we needed to take as a team helped us find the right road. In every case, dedication and hard work are key. Families, schools, and therapists must work together. There's no "magic pill," no shortcut around it.

A Brief Assessment

If my discussion of the communication challenges of boys has validated your concern about your own son or another boy, use the following three checklists to make a more focused assessment. Each checklist reflects a different sphere of communication that shapes social development. These checklists are not a substitute for psychological tests and are intended only to help you sort out your concerns. For simplicity's sake, each checklist is limited to twelve questions. In general, if you find yourself checking more than a few items on any list, there is a strong likelihood that the boy in question could benefit from some family or school intervention to shore up his communication and related social skills.

Has Poor Communication Become a Liability for My Son's Social and Emotional Development?

Does he becomes uneasy when asked opinions or thought-provoking questions? ☐

Does he dread "opportunities" for self-expression? ☐

Does he use anger to deflect personal inquiries? ☐

Does he communicate noticeably less than peers during group interaction? ☐

Does he actively avoid having to speak in front of others? ☐

Does he speak so softly his voice is inaudible or sounds monotone? ☐

Is his nonverbal communication (that is, gestures and expressions) out of sync with his words? ☐

Is he embarrassed about his feelings, even within the safety of parent–child communication? ☐

Does he consistently opt for expressing himself physically versus verbally? ☐

Does he avoid eye contact? ☐

Does he have to be in the right mood to communicate? ☐

Does he attribute his communication difficulties to being "stupid"? ☐

■ ■ ■

Are My Son's Communication Challenges Adversely Affecting Family Life?

Are family gatherings punctuated by uncomfortable silences? ☐

Do sibling rivalries stem from miscommunication? ☐

Do you avoid bringing up some subjects you feel he "can't handle"? ☐

Does he consistently "miss the point"? ☐

Do you feel "tuned out" even when discussing something important? ☐

Are you intimidated by his anger? ☐

Are you and your son comfortable being with each other only when the TV is on? ☐

Do you avoid asking important questions so you don't have to deal with the "grief"? ☐

Is he indifferent to the thoughts and feelings of other family members? ☐

Does he isolate himself from other family members? ☐

Is basic social conversation a struggle for him? ☐

Do family conversations unnecessarily become arguments? ☐

■ ■ ■

Does He Lack the Communication Skills Needed to Succeed Socially and Academically in School?

Does he avoid answering questions in class? ☐

Does he have reading or comprehension difficulties? ☐

Does he isolate himself from other students? ☐

Does he ever act out aggressively to compensate for poor verbal problem-solving skills? ☐

Could untreated or undertreated ADHD be interfering with his learning and social interaction? ☐

Is he often ostracized by other students because he "doesn't get it"? ☐

Do his expressive language skills inadequately reflect his intelligence? ☐

Does he always seems out of sync with peers? ☐

Does he rarely say anything meaningful about his school day? ☐

Does he typically give short or one-word answers on oral or written assignments? ☐

Does he take hours to complete homework requiring expressive writing skills? ☐

Does he hesitate to assert himself even when he knows he should say something? ☐

■ ■ ■

Even if you checked many items on these checklists, there is good reason to hope that things will get better. You've taken the time to think and learn about how to help. Keep what you've recorded on these checklists in mind as you deepen your understanding of boys' communication challenges through the next few chapters. Then, when you read about the specific types of social communication challenges discussed in Part II, return to these checklists to clarify your son's difficulties and what type of help he might benefit from.

The Power of Acknowledgment

For most boys, good communication skills are not about status or sounding exemplary to parents and teachers. Instead, being able to communicate effectively opens the door to a more interesting and rewarding social life. Every time I meet with an adult male whose life has been upended by a poor relationship, explosive anger, or deficient parenting skills (among other behavioral problems that plague men in our society), my passion for improving the communication and social skills of boys grows. The price that our society pays for social incompetence is extraordinarily high. Because no one likes to feel incompetent, chronic frustration may turn into withdrawal, isolation, or even rage.

Giving boys the help and permission they need to be expressive is a major contribution to their emotional well-being. This is because being able to express emotions is the path to *congruity*—the degree of similarity between a person's inner experience and outer behavior. Congruity helps us "feel at home" with ourselves, providing reassurance that we are acting in accord with our deepest feelings and beliefs. This concept is entirely strange to a great many boys. In fact, they are often quite invested in doing just the opposite, which is to say learning to hide their feelings.

You may be reading this and thinking of your own child, how he resists or struggles to adequately express what he is thinking or feeling, how he gets angry when you press him to say more, or how frustrated you feel about growing distant as a result of this communication impasse. The boys we'll discuss in this book will, for the most part, probably be highly recognizable within your family, neighborhood, or community. You may have witnessed the strong reactions

these boys can elicit from adults and peers or how they are sometimes ignored; and you may have been puzzled, worried, or tested by
these boys—within the course of a single day. But make no mistake,
your recognition of these boys is the invaluable starting point. Nothing is so healing as to be seen and understood. It is the beginning of
all possibilities.

TWO

Why Words Matter

■ ■ ■

I magine you've enrolled in an art class at a nearby college. You've never had any
particular talent for art, but you've been advised that this course is required to grad-
uate from school and an important step toward fulfilling your life's aspirations. On
the first day of class, the other students are busy preparing their paints, mixing colors in a
way you've never seen before. Everyone around you seems to be excited about the expressive possibilities of paint and canvas, but things look and feel unfamiliar to you. You
see only primary colors on your palette and have no intuition about how to mix the paints,
but you fumble around, unsure of how to begin.

Soon the others are painting; they seem skillful and confident. Anxious and confused, you sit and stare at your canvas, growing more discouraged by the minute. Everyone else is wondering why you aren't getting started, because they're having so much
fun. They don't realize that you have no idea how to paint. You feel self-conscious and at
least a little irritated by their assumptions. When you finally summon the courage to put
some color on your canvas, the teacher remarks that your colors are a bit dull. He suggests that your "blue needs more life" and that your "red is overpowering—your colors
need to be both clarified and toned down." You don't know what this means or how to do
it. You try again, but the other students have already begun to write you off as untal-
ented.

Increasingly aggravated, you can't define what you're doing wrong. What you do
know is that you've gone from hopeful to dejected faster than you thought possible.
Eventually, the emotional risk of attending class becomes too high—you hate feeling
dumb. You start skipping class and isolating yourself from other students. You think to
yourself, "Who cares about painting anyhow?" and start looking around for other students who also struggle with art, because they make you feel far less self-conscious.

You have discovered the frustration experienced by a boy of few words.

Words are the colors that capture our most important thoughts
and feelings. Although we use thousands of words in a single day,

most of them are chosen relatively unconsciously. Because we tend to speak quickly, and because there is a high degree of redundancy in the words we use, most of us are on autopilot when it comes to word choice. But that doesn't lessen the impact those words will have in our lives and in the lives of those with whom we interact. Words are fundamental to the formation of relationships and deserve far more respect than they are given in day-to-day communication. In fact, we usually take words for granted, except when we "can't find the right word" or when we are in a situation where our words could have significant consequences. At such important or stressful times, most of us have been taught to "choose our words carefully," anticipating how our words will sound to the listener.

Our word choices are also shaped by circumstances, including the particular relationship we have with the person with whom we're communicating. Most of us would address a judge differently from the way we banter with a co-worker. We probably even talk differently to some colleagues as compared with others because we know or trust them more. Such judgments and decisions are a natural part of communication in our life. They require sensitivity to others and an appreciation of social dynamics. Yet the language of many boys lacks awareness of these dynamics, reduced to such basic forms that meaning and expression are lost. Without knowing it, many boys use language in a way that can be detrimental to their social development. The no-frills status of many boys' communication skills should concern us. If words are the currency of most interpersonal exchange, we might reasonably wonder if we are raising a generation of boys on the verge of social bankruptcy.

> ■ ■ ■
>
> When we see boys' anger, we need to look deeper than its outward manifestations. So often, the pouting four-year-old, the socially disruptive eight-year-old, or the disgruntled fourteen-year-old loner is frustrated by an inability to grasp verbal solutions to interpersonal conflicts. Our job as parents is to help them find those words, modeling the phrases they can use to socially connect in constructive ways. "Do you need to tell me you're sorry so we can feel friendly again?" "Maybe if you let him know how much you admire him, he will talk to you." "I think your friends miss you, and they need to know you miss them too."

Some of the psychologically important tasks we use words for include coping with conflict, self-expression, managing stress, and shaping life's most important and, we hope, long-lasting relationships. Look carefully at that list and you'll see that it includes some of the most essential building blocks of psychological well-being. Now imagine someone who doesn't have command of words—stressed out, burdened with conflict, isolated, and potentially explosive.

Language helps us transform emotions into something more tangible, something we can consider or modify. We literally use language to think through the things that happen to us. Experiences are defined and organized in our minds by the words that describe them. The development of our vocabularies makes a big difference in how well we will cope with the challenges life presents. Language helps us mediate our experiences, putting the inevitable adversity and complexity of life into perspective.

The challenge that boys face is to develop sufficient breadth and depth in their social and emotional vocabularies. The breadth of a vocabulary is reflected by the extent of a person's word knowledge, while the depth is reflected by one's appreciation of word meaning and *verbal dexterity*—the ability to apply words effectively and quickly in different situations. Naturally, the expectations we hold for our sons are informed by their age, but even when they are toddlers we should begin helping boys increase both the depth and breadth of their vocabularies.

There are boys who have a sophisticated vocabulary for certain kinds of words. Perhaps they can name every Yu-Gi-Oh! cartoon character and all components of the fantasy world those characters in-

> ■ ■ ■
> You can help even a prereader expand his vocabulary by using lots of synonyms when you talk, especially about emotions: "I'm so *happy* that Grandma is coming to visit. I'm *thrilled!*" "Wouldn't an ice cream cone be *tasty* right now? I think it would be *scrumptious*." "Are you *excited* about going to the zoo? I am—I'm *ecstatic!*"

habit. Other boys know how to build websites or the current lingo for skateboard tricks, but that doesn't equate to being a good communicator. (Note that these examples tend to be vocabularies for things and ideas related to the realms of fantasy, technology, and kinesthetics—activities involving movement.) Boys can become very excited about their interests, and when that excitement gets expressed verbally, strong opinions may follow. Sometimes, however,

■ ■ ■

MOTHER: How was school today?

SON: It sucked.

FATHER: So what are you going to do about these kids who are picking on you?

SON: I don't know, just deal with it.

These kinds of expressions often indicate problems with breadth and depth of expressive vocabulary. When you hear these kinds of statements, consider the possibility that your son's primary problem may be that he doesn't know how to tell you what he feels or thinks. It may help guide the way you respond to him.

hyperbole is mistaken for depth, and strong opinions may be an attempt to divert attention away from more complex thoughts and feelings.

Noah: Learning to Use Words to Understand His Own Emotions

The mother of nine-year-old Noah complained that he was always either angry or quiet. Anyone who met Noah would immediately get the impression that he had a high degree of confidence in expressing his thoughts about things. Noah did not hesitate to describe how he felt about his teacher or what he thought of his family, particularly his father, with whom he had been angry for the better part of two years due to a difficult divorce.

Noah's willingness to talk and be assertive were strengths. At the same time, his success in relating to others was diminished by an inability to participate in more personal, private communication or acknowledge difficult feelings. When I asked Noah if he was having any trouble in his life from being angry, he scowled and turned his head to deflect my inquiry. A long moment of silence passed, and I asked again, but now Noah was frustrated. I could feel his resistance digging in as he responded with "No, not if other people leave me alone." His statement had captured the essence of his social conundrum. Noah didn't know how to be close to someone without escalating his emotions. Getting to know Noah better, I noticed that he often spoke impulsively and that his words were often ill considered.

Sometimes he seemed to enjoy hearing himself make witty or rude remarks. He was more relaxed and talkative when he could dictate the topic or ask the questions. Noah's anger was triggered when he was asked questions that required self-awareness, the relating of emotions to experiences, or involved ambiguous situations without clear "black or white" answers.

Noah's mother and I put together a plan to help him verbalize his feelings about his parents' divorce. This is a difficult task for most children but was particularly hard for Noah. After we had collaborated on this goal for a few months, Noah's mother said, "We were driving to swim practice and talking about his father. I told Noah that I knew all the changes had been hard for him and I loved him. He was very quiet, and I was waiting for some type of complaint or rejection. But he said, 'Sometimes I get mad because I wish I could make you and Dad like each other again.' I think I knew he had felt that all along, but it was a big step for *him* to know he felt that—to put it into words like that. It was like the wall between us was starting to come down, at least a little bit."

In that moment Noah had been able to convey a sense of loss and sadness. The words "I wish" were important, because they implied an objective understanding of his personal, subjective desire (for his parents to "like each other"). He was able to relate how this experience contributed to the way he felt and behaved.

This is how children use language to think through the things that happen to them. Words help them define and clarify their experiences. The measure of our success in life is not whether we have problems or face challenges, because we all do. Our success is measured by how well we manage or cope with our challenges. Boys who learn to use language to understand their experiences are better equipped to accurately identify their emotions and thus less likely to rely on the common male default of undifferentiated anger. Although Noah's circumstance had not changed, his "wish" suggested that he had clarified what he wanted, knew what upset him, and learned to convey this to his mother in a way likely to elicit a supportive response.

As individuals, we use words to capture nuances of personal experience and form the thoughts that help us define who we are. We can effectively use words as symbols or representations of different states of mind. When you think about it, words are a kind of shorthand that quickly captures a feeling or an idea in a way that allows it to be communicated efficiently to others. Most people feel a sense of satisfaction when they find just the right words to convey their thoughts or experiences. We correctly sense that the right words will give our thoughts or experiences a better chance of being understood or appreciated accurately.

And if that important social benefit isn't enough, we can be further encouraged that when we find just the right words to express ourselves, our thoughts and feelings also become clearer to us. Socially, words wind their way through our lives, making up an intricate web that binds

> ■ ■ ■
> Words matter because they help boys define who they are.

us to each other. Your own recollections are testament to how words link the past with the present. Our memories are repositories of the important, impactful words we have heard over the course of our lives—the way our father described how we ride a bike, a compliment given by a teacher about our writing skills, the critical assessment of a peer about how we look, and so on. Long after the last echo of a word can be heard, its meaning resonates deep within us. We must make peace with the words we carry within us, and remember we are responsible for the words we impart to the minds of others.

"I Noticed You Hardly Say Anything—Do You Think We Could Hang Out?"

Even when they don't say so, boys notice communication differences among peers. They sense when their own expressive language skills don't measure up, and by the time they've reached the third or fourth grade, most boys have selected their peer groups based largely on their verbal and social ability. Just as boys who are uncoordinated aren't generally drawn to athletic kids (and aren't always welcomed by them, either), boys lacking verbal skills tend to isolate themselves from their more articulate peers. This schism, and its psychological effects, becomes increasingly apparent in middle school and high school. As we'll see in Part II, boys may cope with this through aggression, anxiety, or withdrawal.

Unfortunately, hanging around with boys with similar communication challenges only distances our sons even further from positive communication influences. And it's not as though those positive influences abound in the first place these days. One reason so many boys lack good language skills is that they are rarely exposed to these skills by important social influences in their lives. When was the last time you heard intelligible syntax or an expanded vocabulary from a popular song, cartoon, or electronic game? (I'm not denying the creativity and expressiveness of these media—but consider the norm marketed to boys.) Instead, the language learning centers of their brains receive a steady barrage of disjointed, fragmented communication infused with marginal syntax and, frequently, devoid of complete thoughts. Even better-quality children's television sometimes overlooks the need to communicate thoughts in complete sentences.

The situation is further complicated by the extraordinarily compelling power of images and their use in almost all forms of communication relevant to children. Imagine if you were taught to walk with crutches—your muscles would be weak and your legs might not function as you would hope. Constantly linking images with words can diminish our ability to use words alone to express ideas.

In a few generations we've gone from listening to radio shows to television accessing over one hundred cable channels, to now desiring elaborate multimedia home entertainment centers. Our senses are steadily dulled by overindulgence in the "drugs" of images and sound. Perhaps this is why so many teachers now find the use of images almost essential to effective learning. In her very insightful book, *Endangered Minds,* education expert Dr. Jane Healy points out that teachers have, sadly, come to expect shortened attention spans and poor listening skills in most students. This situation results in substantially greater difficulty for teachers. They must try to reach children through visual and, especially, auditory learning pathways that tend to be chronically oversaturated and consequently unresponsive to input that isn't highly stimulating. If you recall, much of school is not highly stimulating, at least not in the way that electronic media are. Learning involves lots of repetition, memorization, and incorporation of facts that help scaffold more sophisticated skills and understanding. School is one of the key places where children learn about delaying gratification for the sake of a longer-term goal—promotion to the

■ ■ ■

Words matter because they exercise auditory learning pathways dulled by boys' constant exposure to TV, video games, and computers.

next grade, graduation, or perhaps a career. The changes in how children cognitively process information have not only impacted their learning skills but also have had an acute effect on boys' capacity for social success.

You Are What You Speak

When I meet with boys whose words are muffled, garbled, or sparse, I'm almost always concerned about their emotional well-being. Why? Because I've learned that communication is a type of behavior that *reflects* who we are and who we become—our "self"—but it also *influences* who we are and who we become. This principle of *behavioral bidirectionality* suggests that our actions and our self are in constant dialogue, each shaping the other, whether we are conscious of it or not. For some reason, this fundamental observation about how the mind works was never highlighted during my formal training as a psychologist. Instead, I learned about the principle of behavioral bidirectionality through frustration and a commitment to help some difficult, hard-headed, but otherwise likable teenage boys in rural Pennsylvania.

Beginning one of my first jobs as a therapist, I traveled to several high schools where my responsibility was to counsel "troubled" boys, most of whom also had seriously low self-esteem. Before meeting them, I had decided that my primary strategy would be to provide consistent supportive feedback, commenting on all the positive things I could find in these teenager's lives. Each time we met, I smiled, did my best to project energy and hope, and watched for signs that the boys were changing. I hoped to be something of a role model—that eventually my positive attitude would overcome their negativity and low self-esteem.

This was a considered, well-intentioned approach to making a difference, with only one problem—*it didn't work*. The boys were not willing collaborators despite what I thought was a solid effort on my part. Frustrated, and at times more than a little dejected, I made the long drive home, asking myself what had gone wrong. I was practicing classic counseling skills and sincerely cared about these boys. Still, I had to face the fact that my optimism and hope were not getting through.

Lying awake at night, I wondered what I should do differently.

Gradually, it began to occur to me that maybe I had taken on too much responsibility for making these young men feel better. I had been so busy searching for positives, interpreting their actions and words with an upbeat "spin," that I had not asked them to do any of the hard work that leads to meaningful change. Because of my oversight, I had unintentionally denied them the gift of accomplishment, something boys with low self-esteem desperately need. The boys taught me something I have never forgotten. Offering a positive attitude is not enough to help boys cope with the challenges of childhood and adolescence, nor is it enough to help them transform an impulse toward self-destruction into a momentum toward achievement.

While trying to think creatively about what to do next, I recalled the striking things these boys had told me during their initial assessments. There were stories of all kinds of family conflicts, academic failure, social failure, total disregard for health in the form of substance abuse and sexual promiscuity. In the meetings to follow, I decided to focus more on helping these boys define specific goals, things that mattered to them, and plan actions that would lead to meaningful empowerment. More important, I insisted that they learn to articulate their goals and worked with them to build an "emotional dictionary" that could help modulate negativity through an expanded vocabulary of emotional choices. Many people in the helping professions understand the wisdom of psychologist Abraham Maslow's insight "If you only have a hammer, every problem looks like a nail." In the same sense, if boys can think only in absolutes— like "mad, sad, glad"— they're using sledgehammers even when verbal tools of greater precision are required.

> ▪ ▪ ▪
>
> Words matter because they allow boys to articulate goals and thus give them something to achieve; and achievement is the source of self-esteem.

My experience with these high school boys showed me that building communication skills can encourage healthier self-esteem and that, as self-esteem improves, boys are likely to be more courageous about expressing themselves. This is the principle of bidirectionality at work. A person's mood and outlook follow behavior, and communication is a behavior. The bottom line: As boys improve their ability to express themselves, they open the door to higher levels of confidence and achievement.

Where Do Words Begin?

The seeds of good communication skills are planted while children are still infants and toddlers. The babbling of a two-year-old reflects the sounds that he hears around him, es-

> ■ ■ ■
> Words matter because they are a reflection of your son's emotional well-being and also hold the power to enhance it.

pecially the speech of his primary caregivers. Acquiring language skills draws on a child's ability to detect patterns and rhythms of intonation in his caregiver's speech. During these early years of language development, children are working hard to hear and understand the *forms* of language and speech; for example, how do volume, pitch, tone, and rate of speech convey meaning, such as a sense of urgency? How can babbling or single-word utterances be combined with a gesture to add emphasis or direct a parent's attention? The play of young children is often infused with attempts to mimic the sounds they hear and the gestures they observe in everyday life. An important aspect of play is learning how to apply vocal expression to different contexts. Imaginative play offers children a chance to explore a wide range of communication styles, encompassing a spectrum of possible emotions.

During the toddler years, the rhythms, tones, and patterns of language become increasingly associated with emotional states. The link between the sounds or patterns of communication and particular emotions is reinforced. Three- and four-year-old children are rapidly assimilating information about how to convey their feelings and, as a result, are able to use verbal and nonverbal communication to express emotions more reflexively. The development of these skills can be so dynamic that you see changes in your child from one day to the next! This is an extraordinarily important process for two reasons. First, these associations may stay with a child for a lifetime. The expressive choices your son discovers as a toddler are very likely to inform his expressive style as an adolescent and adult. If you watch a video of your ten-year-old, and compare it to one from when he was four, I think you'll see exactly what I mean.

Second, learning to use communication as a vehicle for emotional expression contributes to learning that words can signify, or act as symbols for, feelings. Of course, children don't think of words this way, and are years from being able to appreciate the concept that language is a symbol system. But as children gain a larger and more specific vocabulary for emotions, they can certainly appreciate the advantages of being able to more clearly express themselves. Parents play a significant role in helping their young sons develop the symbols (words) they will need to represent the range of feelings they will undoubtedly have. Even before we introduce words to children, we see that they associate objects, like stuffed animals or toys, with different emotional states. I'm often struck by how young boys will use toy trucks and cars to represent different kinds of emotions. One truck might be thought of as good, while another is cast as a bad truck within the context of a boy's play. If you listen closely, you'll hear that the rumble these trucks make, by way of your son's presymbolic (preword) vocalizations, are decidedly different. Can you hear the difference between a happy and an angry rumble?

The important thing to remember is that the play of infants and toddlers helps set the stage for the use of words as an efficient and more specific way to communicate. As gestures and words are linked to visible and audible expressions of emotion by a child's parent or caregiver, he learns to make those skills a part of his own emotional vocabulary. Although learning to do this is a natural part of language acquisition for most children, boys can benefit from some extra help and coaching at this critical rung on the emotional development ladder. Boys whose vocabulary for emotions has both breadth and depth are more likely to be both more comfortable expressing their feelings and more attuned to the feelings they have. We will be discussing specific strategies for helping younger boys gain these communication skills in various ways in Chapter 9.

Overall, a child's sensitivity to the expressive capacities of language, and ability to use that sensitivity, is the foundation of social awareness. This type of awareness is sometimes called *social intelligence*. In a world where communication is our passport to social involvement, boys who cannot express themselves are at risk for feelings of inadequacy and disconnection. Being actively involved in building your son's vocabulary is a major contribution to his social and emotional well-being. However, not all boys are fully prepared to take advantage of the effort parents apply toward helping them become better social communicators. As we've already seen, boys are "wired" differently than girls, and are also somewhat more vulnerable to neurodevelopmental challenges. Although this should not stop us from modeling the sounds and tools of communication, sometimes we need to be more strategic, thinking about how to respond to the unique challenges that boys present.

> ■ ■ ■
>
> Words matter because they are ultimately your son's passport to social connection, whether that translates in adulthood to getting along with co-workers, forming rich personal relationships, or feeling a general sense of community with others.

Consider Derek, a six-year-old boy referred to me because he was exceptionally nonverbal. When I first met Derek, he was lying on the floor of my waiting room, mumbling about wanting to go home. His voice was barely audible and he made no eye contact. His parents looked both embarrassed and annoyed. They said they didn't understand Derek's lack of interest in communication and social interaction in general. Derek was an only child, and although they had no point of comparison, his parents felt they had made an honest effort at giving him good verbal skills. They had read to him often, engaged in communicative play using his favorite toys, and made a point of speaking together in a "teaching" way at home. At first they had wondered if Derek's difficulties were related to talking to adults, but as he began school they saw the same behaviors around peers. With classmates, Derek's speech was louder, and his actions more animated, but his overall use of language was still sparse.

> ■ ■ ■
>
> Boys tend to avoid pursuing skills that don't come naturally, because they want to feel, and appear, confident and invulnerable. If we can help boys realize they can master the basics of social communication, their motivation to develop these skills increases exponentially. When your son extends a warm greeting, remembers to ask about your day, or empathizes with a friend, let him know that you appreciate his thoughtfulness. Your own interest in and enthusiasm for these skills is an important yardstick for boys in measuring their worth.

During our second meeting, Derek expressed his interest in the toys and games in my office, although he did so nonverbally by assertively taking toys off their shelves and making a space on the floor to play. His parents prompted him to "ask first," but Derek was undeterred. He did not seem to be a child lacking confidence or awareness about what he liked to do. I interpreted these traits as strengths on which we might eventually build better social communication skills. Getting to that point would be the hard part.

As for many boys of few words, questions made Derek uncomfortable. It was not that he had something to hide, but finding the words to provide a response was difficult and awkward for him. I could see Derek working hard to generate the words and phrases he needed to reply to me, but the difficulty made him tired and bored, and he often gave up or said something completely off-task.

As I evaluated Derek in more depth, it became clear that he had learning differences that put him at a distinct disadvantage when it came to acquiring and using expressive language. Psychoeducational testing indicated a significant problem with the auditory discrimination of different word sounds, commonly called *phonological awareness.* This type of problem is often a significant obstacle to the development of reading skills, as well as social development. Derek's discomfort with language on multiple levels made him a classic boy of few words, having difficulty with verbal expression, reading challenges, and poor interpersonal awareness. Fortunately, Derek had not developed any overt signs of aggression, a common fourth pillar where reading and communication deficits are concerned.

In addition to seeking extra support from a reading skills specialist, I recommended that Derek's parents work with me to develop guided-play techniques that would both interest Derek and make communication the focal point of his interaction with them. The very first ingredient was to apply lots of praise and encouragement whenever Derek made even modest attempts at expressing himself. In addition, his parents began coaching him to be prepared for situations in which he would be expected to communicate socially—such as when visiting my office or going to school. Derek's parents learned to help him practice for these situations by talking through what he might say, modeling vocal expression to indicate emotion and emphasis. This probably resulted in some funny-sounding conversations in the car on the way to school or appointments, but it was an important step toward helping Derek hear the way social communication should sound.

In Derek's case his natural competitiveness and desire for parental approval were valuable "hooks" in getting him to change his outlook on social communication. When boys begin to realize they can do something well that they had previously assigned to the "danger zone," their motivation to work on that problem increases substantially. Our work as parents lies in getting boys to see that they can be good at things that don't necessarily come automatically.

Public and Private Talk

To fully appreciate the communication patterns of males, we need to explore a striking difference between their verbal output in public versus private settings. To be more specific, research over the past thirty years indicates that males tend to be much more verbal in public than they are in private. This phenomenon is at least partially related to males perceiving public environments as a context for social competition, and thus a more engaging forum for communication. Among females, patterns of communication are exactly opposite, with much more talk occurring in private, personal relationships. This gender-based difference in communication reflects other behavioral and psychological differences between males and females as well. It also speaks to the social and cultural roles males and females have traditionally adopted.

Although research data pertaining to this communication difference focus on men rather than boys, if you look closely at the boys in your own life I think you will see a similar pattern. Boys whose expressiveness can hardly be contained at Little League baseball games, lining up for the school bus, or holding court in the school cafeteria are suddenly quiet when asked to communicate one-to-one. In smaller, more personal settings, boys seem to lose motivation for making themselves heard. Rather than engaging, they are often looking for an exit strategy.

When we consider this phenomenon with respect to vocabulary, we should recognize that word knowledge also contributes to boys being more verbal in public than in private. This is because despite the auditory disadvantages of boys that we discussed in the previous chapter, their brains are magnets for the language of conquest and competition. As I was writing this very chapter, I took a break to take my son to the playground, where he joined

▪ ▪ ▪

Do men or women talk more?
In part, the answer lies in where the conversation takes place. Males tend to be more verbal in public domains; females tend to speak more in private, personal situations. Your son may be the team chatterbox but at a loss for words at the dinner table. Your daughter may talk on the phone for hours but hesitate to speak her mind in a group. The times and places we use our words reflect important aspects of our social development.

several other boys in the kind of lively play they love. I will concede that my writing had sensitized me to what I was hearing, but amid the shouts and cries I recorded the following statements verbatim: "You will never beat me," "I'm the king," "Ha-ha, you can't catch me now," "I'll crush you with my claw," "My swing can go higher," and my personal favorite, "You can't stand up to my magic." These are more than examples of the public language of children. This is the socially competitive language of boys who use play to enact the psychological dramas that shape their social interaction.

In many cases, the public communication of boys contrasts starkly with their grasp and use of words in private. My point is not that we can, or even should, strive to get boys to follow the communication pattern of girls, only that a large number of boys would benefit from more balance in where, when, and how they communicate. If communication comes easily only when it's time to compete, boys will logically seek out competition to experience the pleasure of self-expression. What of the words that define different kinds of relationships? When will boys develop an ear for the vocabularies of cooperation, conscience, and consideration? The words that make up these vocabularies are the words that will enable our sons to succeed as they mature and become part of new groups at school and work.

> ▪ ▪ ▪
> Words matter because they give boys a vocabulary for succeeding in groups at school and later at work—a vocabulary they might lack if left to their own preferences to express themselves largely in competition.

Does He Hear Some Words Better Than Others?

Not all words are created equal. We have heightened sensitivity to the words and language that speak to our individual lives. These are the words that boys absorb and remember best, and these are the words that boys so often make the centerpiece of their personal mythology. Because boys are individuals, attracted to a wide variety of interests and activities, it's hard to predict where they will hear the words that will captivate their imaginations—or the words that help them define themselves. For a nine-year-old, these words may be derived from a favorite cartoon, yet even among nine-year-olds one boy longs to emulate the brainy heroism of "Jimmy Neutron, Boy Genius," while another prefers the absurd wit of "Sponge Bob's" aquatic world. For a fifteen-year-old, the words of greatest impact more likely come from music and the colloquial language of peers. The words that speak to an adolescent seat themselves deep within his verbal consciousness, and you probably hear the same words and phrases over and over again as teenage boys apply them stylistically to their conversational speech.

It can be hard to understand or appreciate why our sons are so attracted to certain kinds of words or language. Our understanding will be aided if we remember that a person's language and communication choices reflect the person and emotions within. Not long ago, I read about a marketing company that discovered that when it played more edgy, "anxious" jazz on its clients' telephone systems, it had fewer hang-ups than when it played slow, lilting classical music. The discovery was quite surprising to the company's executives, who had long assumed that calm music would soothe the agitation of having to wait to speak with a "real person." However, it seemed that callers preferred to hear music more congruent with their internal state. When callers heard edgy jazz, their emotions (in this case irritable impatience while waiting for the next customer service representative) were being reflected and anchored effectively. Net result: Callers were much less likely to turn away from music that spoke to the immediacy of their emotional experience. This illustration underscores why it is particularly important to pay attention to the music that speaks to our sons, including the lyrics that become core elements of their everyday speech. Listening deeply to your son can be a wonderful starting point for the type of dialogue you hope for, one in which you move

▪ ▪ ▪

Listen closely to the words that speak to your son, whether in song lyrics or seemingly insignificant banter with friends.

beyond superficialities to connect with your son's deeper ways of understanding and expressing himself.

As we've already seen, words are symbols, and as boys reach adolescence, words become symbols for increasingly complex ideas and emotional states. Experimenting with forms of expression that their parents don't approve of is an age-old rite of passage for adolescents. So if your son is listening to "gangsta" rap, you may wonder whether it reflects antisocial feelings within him or a fascination with the dynamics of power and the tension between good and evil. In some respects, this music is a relatively safe way to explore and understand the dual nature of oneself—flirting with the taboo thoughts and impulses that live within all of us. (Every generation has its rebel songs. Not long ago I read an interview with the late, great country singer Johnny Cash. He noted that the line that always got the biggest rise from his audience was "I shot a man in Memphis, just to watch him die." The coldness of that line spoke to an earlier generation's fascination with an enduring aspect of being human—curiosity about humanity's "dark side.") Trying to argue with an adolescent about the music he likes is an exercise in frustration because his appreciation of music has far less to do with taste than the search for symbols. Our sons are justifiably excited when they discover symbols for the developmental processes that dominate their life and self-awareness. Adopting a confrontational, authoritarian stance with boys will only make the words more powerful. Instead, asking your son to explain the lyrics and what they evoke in him could lead to a more enlightening and productive conversation. This is the most important reason we should be aware of the words that speak to our sons—so that we can effectively maintain verbal contact.

Our ability to communicate with boys provides needed reassurance and helps to compensate at least somewhat for their hesitancy to initiate communication with us. Yet open communication also serves another, equally important function—helping our sons avoid the descent into self-absorption. When boys lose interest in learning new things, when they stop making an effort to cross bridges into the lives of others, and when they become indifferent to the words and actions of even the people who know them best, we have a significant problem on our hands. Self-absorbed boys can give you the impression that they are in a type of trance, thinking and feeling within a private reality we cannot access. Sometimes boys shut down for lack of a better alternative. It simply feels easier to withdraw into oneself than struggle with the demands of life.

■ ■ ■

Words matter because they break down the wall of self-absorption that threatens to build itself around our sons.

Evan

One morning, the principal of a small high school called me. A very worried ninth-grade girl had come to see her. She said that another student, named Evan, had threatened to hurt himself. Evan reportedly had told the girl that she could have his music, scores that he had written himself, because he wouldn't need them anymore.

The principal conveyed her belief that Evan was both intelligent and creative, but had trouble relating to peers. Evan's parents had transferred him to the school from a larger public high school. They felt that a small school, one that could challenge Evan academically and could support his interest in computers and music, would be perfect. He was close to finishing his junior year at his new school, and the news of what he had said was a surprise to everyone.

The school had contacted Evan's parents, advising them to take him to a nearby hospital for evaluation. The principal had just received a call from Evan's father, who was upset because he and Evan had been sitting around the hospital for several hours, without a decision as to whether Evan would be admitted. In turn, the principal called me to see if I might help get the situation resolved. She said, "We want to keep him safe, but at the same time, we don't want to see him hospitalized if it turns out that the girl was being a little dramatic or misunderstood him."

Following a conversation with the doctor on call at the emergency room, it was agreed that the hospital would release Evan, but with the caveat that he see a therapist and return to the hospital if he could not contract to keep himself safe. I met Evan, at 9:00 P.M. that evening, escorted by his worried and exasperated parents. He was a thin, serious-looking boy with straight, dark hair just long enough to be pulled back into a ponytail. He wore silver glasses, a T-shirt printed with musical notes, and jeans.

"Evan," I said, "it's nice to meet you. I guess you've had a pretty intense day?"

His father quickly interjected, "We need some answers. *He* won't tell us anything."

Evan's mother replied, "It doesn't seem like he knows what to say. I keep asking him what's going on. Is he trying to hurt us? What are we supposed to do?"

Despite the irritation in their voices, there was no doubt their world had been turned upside down by the day's events. Clearly, this constituted a family crisis, but it was also apparent that it would be helpful to give Evan some space to be heard alone. I asked his parents to give me a chance to meet with Evan privately, and I made sure to let Evan hear me express assurance to his parents that we could resolve whatever was troubling him. Given their level of anxiety, I knew this would be comforting to his parents, but I also feel it is important for kids who may be very confused about their own feelings to encounter someone who can normalize that confusion and who is confident about improving the situation.

Over the course of the next hour, Evan's story began taking shape. He had been at the school since his sophomore year. The classes were very small and students could essentially design their own curriculum, setting goals and then participating in group meetings to report on their progress. Evan had three passions: computers, music, and martial arts. He had developed an interesting project, translating some of the movements from karate into musical notes. For example, a specific type of kick might translate to the musical note "C"; therefore a certain sequence of moves might be translated as "C, C-flat, E," and so on. These sequences would be programmed into the computer and he would synthesize music from them.

The previous week, Evan had to present his idea to a group at school. His teacher had been very encouraging, but some of the kids had asked him how this would make good music. One girl had suggested that he write the music first and then adapt the karate moves to the music. This had infuriated Evan; he was emphatic that there was a particular sequence to the karate moves and that he could not change the order. Isolating himself from peers, he continued to ruminate about the "stupid suggestion" and his rage grew steadily over the course of the week, spiraling into self-doubt, dejection, and eventually, dramatic thoughts and self-destructive impulses. Evan wanted the girl who made the suggestion to understand and admire him, and he took her comment as a rejection of himself and his work. He'd given the girl his project notebook with his music score, and said he wouldn't live to hear it played.

"What did you mean by that?" I asked.

"I don't know," said Evan.

"Did you plan to hurt yourself?"

"I don't know. I just hate everything right now," he said. "What does it matter? Nobody gets it."

"Does anybody get you?" I asked.

"I don't know, should they?" Evan replied.

■ ■ ■
When boys answer questions with other questions, their emotional defenses have been activated.

My radar told me my question had hit home and Evan was feeling vulnerable.

Evan was typical of many boys of few words. He was attracted to activities and interests where there are formulas and structure, mathematical rules that could help him wade through an otherwise confusing world of verbal nuance, shifting perspectives, diverse groups. Life becomes more difficult for such boys when they enter adolescence. In high school, tasks require more sophisticated problem solving, the ability to integrate information from multiple sources and make stylistic and ethical judgments. I was most interested in Evan's attraction to music. He was fascinated by the structural dynamics of music and the elegance of chords, tones, and sequences. He fantasized about creating a musical formula to describe different feelings. His major problem was that he couldn't make music that sounded good to people.

So over the course of my work with Evan we approached his emotional illiteracy through the language of music. Evan wanted to take a mechanistic approach. He wanted to know which musical phrases sounded sad and which ones sounded happy to others. His goal was to have a set of musical algorithms for emotions. I could sense how if this were possible, his perceived sense of safety, relative to emotions, would improve. Evan expressed the idea intellectually, but the sincerity of his quest was palpable.

It was obvious that my best chance at connecting with Evan was through his music. Watching someone listen to his music was very satisfying to Evan, the closest he ever got to a true smile. He would bring in his compositions recorded on a compact disc, which could be played on my office computer. Evan would narrate these listening sessions with indications of what emotions he was trying to represent. After several sessions, I asked him why he never wrote any lyrics to his music. The question surprised him, seeming to strike him as almost illogical.

"I don't know, I just never thought about it," he replied.

We agreed that music would continue to be the cornerstone of our meetings as long as he started the process of writing lyrics. I told him it was okay to express anything—even his confusion about *what* to express. He wrote his lyrics in his notebook, and preferred that I read them silently while we listened to his music. To read the lyrics over the course of several months was to see a remarkable journey of self-exploration. There were numerous ups and downs, moments of clarity and confusion, yet an overriding sense that Evan was moving closer to a better understanding of himself. I began to see that Evan himself felt better when he could translate his musical intentions into words.

My work with Evan revealed that he did have emotions and was at least somewhat motivated to express them. When free of disabling anxiety and self-consciousness, Evan's expressive skills were significantly better. As Evan grew more accepting of himself, I could sense his hope that maybe he was not doomed to the life sentence of social and emotional isolation he feared.

Evan is now in college, and I get an occasional e-mail from him to let me know how he's doing. He and his parents strategized about where he should attend college and decided that an arts-oriented university would be a good fit academically and would also provide a social network of individuals tuned in to Evan's "frequency" of communication. He tells me he's on the dean's list and that he plays keyboard for a band—and they've used one of his songs. He e-mailed the lyrics, and although he didn't tell me outright, I suspect he wanted me to know he has learned something about love.

> *When I let you see me*
> *Then you know*
> *Come on and find me*
> *Then we'll go*
> *If it's love we're feeling*
> *Let it flow*
> *Let it show.*
> —Lyrics from Evan's song, "The Key"

Communication Is at the Root of Community

Words have a tremendous impact on the course of human relationships. They are powerful tools in the minds of boys who know how to use them. Words can be used for good or bad, socially or antisocially. As parents, mentors, or teachers, our job is to help boys learn the code of social communication and to appreciate how their lives and relationships can be transformed positively by language. To be sure, this is an ambitious undertaking and must be guided by a strong sense of purpose. I believe we can find that sense of purpose in our own conscience and the legacy we want to impart to our children.

Boys without the right words cannot adequately know themselves or understand and relate to others. Are we willing to accept their challenges as a preordained limitation, or should we strive to expand their opportunities? How will we teach our sons about the importance of balancing their own needs with those of others? The answer can only be that we must nurture the words that anchor a boy's conscience within a world broader than himself. It is through words that we become known to each other, and it's through words that we form relationships and come to be responsible to each other—that we come to recognize ourselves as part of the human community.

Even if you share my enthusiasm for the potential of boys to contribute to the lives of others, you may justifiably wonder why the job has to be so hard. More specifically, you may wonder why so many boys avoid private communication and why it is so difficult or awkward for them to talk with you. Understanding the psychology of boys is a mandatory step in knowing how to reach them. In the next chapter we'll consider how a boy's mind works when it comes to personal communication. We will need to suspend judgment and open our own minds to experience why boys think and feel as they do.

THREE

Why Doesn't He Talk to Me?

...

When my son was born, the first time I held him he returned my gaze and grasped my finger with his hand. It felt like a miracle, yet it's an experience known to millions of parents, signaling that a lifetime of communication between parent and child has begun. Especially in our child's earliest years, we are captivated by his ability to learn, enchanted by his first words, and intrigued by his ideas. We listen to him closely, trusting that his words are a barometer of his psychological and social development. We're proud when he learns to introduce himself, surprised he can name all the dinosaurs, and dismayed by his fascination with "bad" words. Primarily, we welcome our child's communication. His first instances of self-expression help us get to know him; even in early infancy we observe his mannerisms and reactions to get clues about his personality and temperament. We talk about boys who are "wild" and boys who are sensitive, notice that one child had a sense of humor from early on, and appreciate the serious focus of another. As a child grows, his communication becomes more sophisticated and interactive. We get to know him better—and he gets to know us, learning how words can navigate relationships.

It's both amusing and alarming to hear your four-year-old advise you to "take it easy" in the midst of your morning rush to leave the house on time or observe that he knows you just can't resist it when he smiles a special way and says "please." At the deepest levels of our being, we sense that communication is the pathway to the emotional connections that strengthen family relationships. Through the rhythms of language, parents and children establish the cadence of family life. We listen for these familiar rhythms as a sign of reassurance that all is well within our families. Every family has its own unique sound and private language. Some families buzz and bustle, everyone talking at once. Others murmur more quietly, perhaps breaking the surface with a thoughtful observation or inside joke. Whatever our style, communication is the means by which we teach and come to understand our children. Through communication we form the deep, reciprocal relationships that are life's reward.

But what are we supposed to think if our son is less than enthusiastic about our attempts to build connection? How should we interpret a boy's choice not to communicate or to limit communication to only the most practical, mundane aspects of daily life? What do we do when the baby we held in our arms now uses sharp and painful words, fending off our attempts to reach him? And how is it that boys who have generally been emotionally open and communicative through the first decade of life so often become guarded and defensive in their second decade?

Experiencing a communication withdrawal in our sons is both perplexing and frustrating, complicated by having come to rely on his words as a window to his psychological world. (This can be particularly difficult for mothers, who by necessity must bridge both a generation *and* a gender gap.) After all, talking is one of the most fundamental ways that people relate to each other. It seems reasonable for parents to expect their sons to speak with them in a way that reflects mutual respect and basic involvement in family life. Communication expresses social interest, and when our sons don't talk to us it can feel as though they are disinterested or somehow pulling away or rejecting us. The child who for years was inseparable, who had so many questions and needed to tell us everything, may suddenly feel like someone we don't know or understand. Even worse, he can feel like someone who doesn't want to know us. My experience in working with families has shown me how deeply worrisome this situation can be. Parents can feel the sting of apparent disinterest yet also be guided by an instinctive inner voice that tells them their sons do indeed need them. As parents, we must sometimes rely on the strength of that voice to sustain our love and effort—even when boys may appear to be working diligently to convince us that our efforts are in vain.

We can also rely on a deep understanding of the practical and psychological factors that might be causing our sons to be less communicative than we'd like. As we consider these factors, it's important to remember that when we are talking about a group as broad as males, manifestations of masculinity are as varied as individual boys and men. Your own son is a unique person whose personality and behavior represent a complex combination of genetics, learning, *and* gender. In fact, your acknowledgment of his uniqueness is essential to your getting through to him, perceiving his reality, and, eventually, helping him appreciate yours.

Your reality, however, might differ depending on whether you're a mother or a father. Both mothers and fathers get concerned when their sons don't communicate, but because of different gender perspectives, they often understand communication problems from complementary perspectives. If you can sustain a constructive discussion of those perspectives, you have the foundation for an effective parenting team. Acknowledging that your gender shapes how you view your son will help you meet him halfway across the communication divide.

Is It a Phase, a Personality Trait, or a Problem?

Viewing boys' communication in a developmental context, it is often easier to make sense of the *hows* and *whys* that shape their choices and actions. Boys face different developmental challenges at different ages. Communication changes over time as the facts of a boy's life change, both biologically and situationally. Your sensitivity to these changes, and willingness to develop responsive solutions, will have a significant impact on your son's life. A note of caution, however: Recognizing that communication patterns evolve as boys get older is not the same as believing a boy will "just grow out of it." It's not always easy to tell when taking a "wait and see" attitude has outlived its usefulness, so the best policy is usually to check in regularly with a little analysis of what you're seeing.

To start, when you have a concern about your son's communication, ask yourself if his challenges seem out of line with his other abilities. Jean, the mother of 11-year-old Seth, worried because her son would rarely talk to her about his school day. She consistently made an effort to learn about Seth's friends and about the many things she knew he was learning. Seth barely acknowledged her questions, saying only that "school's okay" or "I don't know" whenever

Jean asked questions that required more thought or an opinion. On the positive side, Jean noticed that her son was comfortable among peers and was quite popular when it came to games and sports. Her observations prompted me to ask some questions about Seth's early development.

"How old was he when he walked?" I asked.

"Very young," Jean responded, "at least by ten months."

"And what about talking?"

"That was much later. He didn't start with putting a few words together until he was almost three," she said.

As it turned out, Seth's verbal development had always lagged behind his physical skills. While the lag was initially small, over the course of his life it had become more pronounced. This is because boys like Seth often sense early on that talking is not what they do best. Instead of practicing where they need it most, they divert their attention away from what makes them feel awkwardly self-conscious and toward what comes more easily. Boys learn by trial and error how to strengthen self-esteem. Once they develop a set of beliefs about who they are and what they are and aren't good at, it can be extraordinarily difficult to convince them otherwise.

For boys of all ages, there are levels of communicative ability that are appropriate, but the range is varied. In general, we like to see boys communicating at a level near their peers, in a manner that you can be comfortable with, and in a way that gives them a fair chance of being successful in school and in relationships. We also like to see them developing at roughly the same pace across different developmental domains. So if you have a son like Seth, you don't necessarily have reason to worry, but knowing from the start that his verbal ability lags behind his motor skills can motivate you to pay extra attention to encouraging speech.

Begin to Understand Why by Observing

When you're initially concerned about your son's level of communication, there are a number of things you want to find out:

■ *Do his communication problems stem from disinterest, resistance, or a lack of ability?* How do his communicative abilities contrast with his other areas of development? How do his other physical, moral/social, and intellectual phases of development compare? If you would describe your son's overall behavior as "young for his age," it may be that he hasn't had time or practice to develop appropriate communication skills.

■ *Does his communication change in certain circumstances or in response to different people?* Is the problem being caused by a specific situation or within a specific relationship? Boys can be sociable and witty at a friend's house but quiet and sullen at home. This type of variation in your son's communication often occurs during preadolescence, when boys are more inclined to gravitate toward the influence of peers over family. Yet observing this behavior in your son might also tell you it's time to try communicating on a different "frequency." Have you considered initiating conversations that elicit his opinions or focus on learning more about his interests?

■ *Try changing the way you communicate with him and see if it changes how he responds to you.* Does he need some extra time to process your queries? Does he understand what you're asking? Is he particularly tongue-tied when it comes to discussing his feelings, hopes, fears, and desires? One of the classic techniques used by therapists can also be helpful at home. Bring your discussion with your son into the "here and now." This means asking him how you come across to him. It's easy to get sidetracked into focusing on the content of your message without paying due attention to its form. Don't be afraid to tell your son openly how you would like to be perceived—and please don't get defensive if he tells you something unexpected about your own communication. Great parents follow their own advice!

■ *Ask others in his life about their impressions of his communication, particularly parents or teachers of other boys his age.* A consensus of opinion can validate or relieve concerns. Following a parent–teacher conference, the parents of eight-year-old Hans discovered they were not the only ones perplexed about his intense fascination with Ferris wheels and unwillingness to talk of little else. Their son's teacher helped them make the decision to investigate the issue with a professional.

As parents, our primary concern is to see each boy as an individual and to focus on how his communication is impacted by the broader psychological factors that may shape his life. Some of these factors are best understood as personality traits, while others are better understood as being part of some type of developmental experience, which at least temporarily changes the way boys talk and relate to others. These temporal experiences might include, among other things, family relationships, school changes, transition to the next grade level, new friends or interests, self-esteem changes, onset of puberty, experimentation with rebellion, and the emergence of strong sexual feelings. And this list only scratches the surface! When affected by such developmental experiences, boys can be very talented at fooling parents with signs of apparent indifference. They want us to believe they can handle whatever life throws their way, because generally speaking, that is the message boys believe they are expected to convey to the world—if not by parents, then at least by peers. If you've spent time with boys past the age of twelve, you've seen these signs of indifference in their expressionless faces, defiant or poor eye contact, and related signals of "emotional shutdown." If you're to understand why your son doesn't talk to you, you might have to start by knowing why boys present this image to the world. What motivates them to use these psychological defenses? Once you know the purpose these defenses serve, you can creatively work around them to sustain and enhance communication with your son.

"Real Boys Don't Talk"

There are few things as alarming to most boys, or males of any age for that matter, as the prospect of showing vulnerability, specifically emotional vulnerability. Being vulnerable may help you to be open and responsive, but it also exposes your fears, confusion, or weaknesses. Although females may not be eager to embrace vulnerability either, the fear of vulnerability takes on a significantly different shape in boys and men. For many males, fear of any kind is undesirable, if not unacceptable, and boys learn early in life to shield their fear from others.

Some social scientists and anthropologists have argued that, in part, males are averse to expressing vulnerability due to the behavior-shaping forces of evolution, noting that during earlier times in human history signs of weakness could have threatened a male's chances of survival (such as being more likely to be attacked by rivals or having less access to prospective mates seeking his protection). Broadly stated, according to this evolutionary perspective, vulnerable males were weeded out of the gene pool, while males possessing characteristics of aggression and related traits of invulnerability prospered.

If we look at conflicts in the world today, whether between warring nations or tensions between peer groups in school, we can see the roots of the reflex to suppress vulnerability. The time-honored game of "chicken" is a good example of this reflex, as boys and men test each other on "who will flinch first." Certainly, we all know situations where it's advantageous to appear strong or invulnerable, for safety or success. Unfortunately, many boys are socially reinforced for their ability to withhold signs of emotion. A "poker face" is seen as the face of a warrior, even though stoicism or confrontation is not particularly useful in most modern settings—and is often, in fact, counterproductive.

On the time line of human development, our circumstances have changed more quickly than our genes. Genetically, our sons may still be better programmed to defend against predators than to foster cooperation in a town or an office. There are a lot more of us living on this earth than there were in the Stone Age, and by necessity we need to interact and get along. Our economy is service oriented, meaning we have to talk with other people all the time. It's also information driven, and information demands exchange between one person and the next. When we focus on teaching our sons communication skills, we do this not because it is politically correct or fashionable but because the social and cultural forces of our time require these skills for success and fulfillment. All of this may seem painfully obvious to you. Sadly, it may not be to your son.

Boys do not like to feel unsure of themselves, and they will actively avoid situations and experiences that deflate their self-esteem and sense of competence. Along with a probable genetic contribution to this survival instinct of invulnerability, there are tremendous social forces at play as well. While girls will often express self-doubt or vulnerability as a way to form closer relationships with friends (and also as a way to fend off accusations of vanity or arrogance), boys who admit their worries or confusion are often shamed or punished, especially by peers but sometimes by adults as well. Well-meaning parents may not anticipate the discomfort caused by probing for answers boys are unprepared to provide. For boys, the prospect of sorting out conflicting needs or relating to others in ways that highlight their insecurities is a frightening one. Rather than inviting such experiences as an opportunity to learn, boys are inclined to feel that these "opportunities" are destabilizing emotional experiences, forcing them to confront the most vulnerable aspects of themselves. If you can remember this basic principle—*minimizing vulnerability increases the likelihood of open communication*—you will have taken a strategic step toward effectively relating to boys. Your son has to know that it is safe for him to remove the mask of stoicism, at least with you.

■ ■ ■

When you make your son feel vulnerable—or even at risk of appearing vulnerable—he's likely to clam up. Communication with boys flows more easily when you . . .

- Avoid sarcasm and criticism.
- Express positive interest when he takes the initiative to talk to you; restate his comments so he knows you're listening.
- Talk while you're doing an activity together, rather than sitting down for a formal "talk."
- Avoid "overquestioning."
- Respect his confidentiality (within reasonable limits).
- Acknowledge the skills and abilities he does possess.
- Let him hear and converse with open, articulate men.

"I Don't *Know* How I Feel—So I'd Rather Not Think about It"

Although boys may not consciously choose to avoid self-awareness, they are often hampered by an underdeveloped vocabulary of emotions, a subject we'll get into in more depth in the next chapter. The result is that boys often lack the necessary tools to clarify who they are and what they feel—even to themselves. The idea of "feelings" in general overwhelms boys. Strong emotions detract from boys' sense of self-confidence, because the realm of feelings is inherently more intuitive, with soft edges. Gaining self-awareness requires boys to tolerate emotional ambiguity, at least for a while, as they come to know themselves more deeply. For example, an emotionally aware person might understand that he can feel more than one way about a situation or realize that his emotional response doesn't live up to his ideals about how he should feel. Yet for the majority of boys, crisp thoughts and actions are a far preferable experience. Throughout life, males struggle with experiences over which they have relatively little control. In the many marital therapy sessions I have led, I have seen over and over how difficult it is for men to encounter emotional problems without feeling anxious to rush to a "practical" or "quick" solution. Boys, as well, are much more comfortable dealing with concerns that have clear parameters and harder edges. These are the types of challenges that more naturally invite boys to engage analytical, solution-focused thinking.

In part, this explains why interpersonal communication is difficult for so many boys. This type of communication tends to evolve organically, requiring spontaneity and flexibility—you usually can't plan what you're going to say far in advance; you have to respond to what the other person says in the moment. For many boys, these moments are filled with unbearable pressure. They feel as though they are being stared at and that others are waiting for them to say something smart! Such psychological transitions often mystify boys, who don't easily grasp the cues or "rules" that guide social communication. As frustrated as parents can be in trying to get past this kind of social awkwardness, boys are often equally frustrated, and they will quickly revert to an attitude of anger to show you how they feel about being asked to tread on ground where they feel insecure.

> ■ ■ ■
>
> When teaching a boy to express himself, think of a radio with two dials, one for volume, one for stations. Boys can learn about a variety of intensities in their emotions, or "volumes" (from "I'm annoyed" to "I'm furious"), but they also need to learn how to tune in different stations of emotion, to experience a variety of feelings. Boys don't have to be frozen on the "anger station." They can dial a range of frequencies (from pride to embarrassment, fear to courage) and fine-tune their emotional experiences. But when they're not talking to you, it may be because they don't yet know that.

Boys don't always resist communication out of defiance. Often, they don't actually know what it is they feel or think about something. This is not an easy thing for parents to understand or accept. For adults who take pride in being in touch with themselves, it is almost inconceivable. When I brought up this issue with Julia, the mother of a quiet but otherwise well-adjusted fourteen-year-old, Ryan, she looked incredulous, exclaiming, "How can he be so disconnected?" assuming others were as in touch with their emotional selves as she was. Julia was concerned because Ryan refused to talk about the death of a young cousin. When prompted, Ryan said he felt sad, yet his words somehow lacked feeling, and no amount of prodding could get him to say more. The incident had crystallized the worries Julia had been developing about Ryan for several years. She wondered why he was so much less talkative than his older brother and other boys in their neighborhood. "I alternate between being worried that he's carrying an unbearable weight all by himself and being afraid that he doesn't care as much as I think he should. Sometimes I wonder if he's trying to punish us in some way." It's natural to search for an explanation that relates cause and effect. Not infrequently, misguided expectations lead us to see resistance to communication as an act of revolt, rather than the result of a boy needing more time to fully understand what's going on within himself. When boys are hesitant to talk, there is a high probability that they do not want to reveal their thoughts before they're sure of what they think or feel. In a way, Julia's concern that Ryan didn't feel "deeply enough" hit the mark. It can be very difficult for anyone to face painful emotions and particularly hard for boys who avoid the realm of feelings. One reluctant, but insightful, teenager described his fear this way: "If I think about it too much, it's like standing at the edge of a cliff. I can't stand to look. I just want to back away."

"All I Know Is That I'm Really Mad!"

So often, when boys feel vulnerable, their feelings are transformed into anger. Overall, this is a much more manageable emotion for most boys, who equate expressions of anger with an expression of power—a highly desirable, even coveted, trait for most males. Angry communication is often a boy's first reflex in coping with humiliation or confusion, because expressed anger is a kind of aggression, an attempt to combat very uncomfortable emotions. From an early age, boys learn to use anger to ward off people who may try to penetrate the protective veneer they so masterfully construct to conceal their emotional selves. (If your boy of few words resorts to anger much of the time, be sure to read Chapter 6.) We might justifiably wonder why boys resist communication if it could help them know themselves better. Yet if we remember that the search for self-awareness makes many boys

■ ■ ■

For boys to be self-expressive they have to know how they feel, and so often they don't. Combine that uncertainty with their aversion to feeling doubtful and incompetent—therefore vulnerable—and you have boys who don't talk except to shout and who think that expressing an opinion means "throwing it in your face." Sometimes what appear to be aggressive statements stem from fear or confusion.

uncomfortable, perhaps we can appreciate their hesitation.

In general, boys are much more invested in the world of things and actions than in introspection, seeking mastery through knowledge of systems, how things work, and winning in competition. Our culture celebrates these qualities in boys, and it would be unfair to ask boys to forgo the acknowledgment and approval they crave. If you listen carefully to boys, you will hear this *craving* everywhere. I was recently in a marine supply store and overheard a classic conversation between a boy and his younger sister.

She pointed and said, "What's that? Is that an anchor?"

"Yes it is," he agreed and, apparently wishing to seem authoritative, continued, "It can also be used for hitching to tug boats and as a hook for deep-sea fishing." "Really? How do you know that?" his sister replied, slightly suspicious of this "fish tale."

"Because I'm so smart!" he replied, emphatically.

"Okay, if you're so smart, what's the biggest word *you* know?" she retorted.

"Who cares? That's stupid!" he snapped, changing the subject. "These anchors can also be used as harpoons, you know."

Notice that he asserted his knowledge of how the anchor "worked," and she challenged his language expertise. When we seek to connect with our sons, we can be more successful if we understand their desire to appear confident and knowledgeable. The bravado and cockiness of some boys is their way of asserting "I know how things work. I am clever and competent. I am important. Don't you love and admire me?" When we ask boys to enter territory that is unfamiliar, mutable, or uncomfortable (such as in conversations where boys have to respond off-the-cuff to queries that may not have clear answers, or in situations that are emotionally or morally ambiguous), a "safe" default is anger.

Think of a boy's emotions as a pressure cooker with just one release valve: "I don't know how to express myself, I can't appear weak or confused, but I've got to have relief somehow" . . . kaboom! It's not always obvious to boys that strong, confident men can express themselves in a variety of ways and can safely admit when they don't know something. This understanding must be reinforced at the levels of leadership occupied by parents, teachers, and mentors. These are the people to whom boys look for guidance and from whom they learn how to sculpt their own model of masculinity.

A Boy's Silence Can Mean Different Things

Silence is a powerful tool that boys consciously and unconsciously use to shape the atmosphere of relationships. Silence can be a deviant expression of power, used to convey an attitude of indifference or defiance, or it can grow from intense anxiety and insecurity. When a boy's silence makes us uncomfortable, it's easy to forget ourselves, perhaps pushing harder. There's a difference between the silence that is in and of itself a powerful form of expression and the silence that flows from confusion about what to say or how to say it.

Marla is a very sharp prosecuting attorney I've been seeing as a client on and off for a few years. Although she never brought her son in to see me, her account of her son's silence really resonated with what I often see happening between parents and sons. "I've just always loved to think on my feet, and I'm usually confident about what people really think when they speak—that's my job," she said. "But there's a reason why people don't like it when someone takes the Fifth. You just can't be sure you understand what the silence means. My son really shut down with me following my divorce, and of course I attributed it to the aftereffects. But it went on so long, I knew it had to be something else. It got to the point where I would lie awake trying to analyze the problem, pretending he wasn't my son so I could be more objective. It finally came to me that the moment he opened his mouth and said something more than 'Where's the cereal?'—if he said anything remotely personal—I always responded with a question. And if he answered, I would ask another, and then another, and another. I was cross-examining this kid totally unintentionally. He didn't get that I love him and was worried about him, and I was just trying so hard to be close to him. The poor kid felt like he was getting cross-examined—my own son was taking the Fifth with me! I started putting a dollar in a jar every time I answered him with a question. The first week his allowance was quadrupled, but after that I slowed down. I learned to restate what he had said or just nod and be quiet, to give him time to compose his thoughts. I just had to pull back a little. The impact was remarkable."

> ■ ■ ■
>
> Instead of repeating your question when your son doesn't answer, come back to it later or try asking the question with a softer tone, or when you and your son are engaged in an activity together. He will feel more relaxed to be doing something, which in turn might allow the flow of thoughts and words to come more easily.

The silence of boys can hang heavy in the air, or it can go unnoticed. Sometimes boys are selectively silent, giving you ample information about externals like hobbies, sports, games, and television, but staying well clear of more personal matters. So skilled are some boys at turning the conversation away from anything revealing or relational, it can be difficult to put your finger on what's missing. And sometimes people can willfully misinterpret "small talk," hoping it is a precursor to something more. Dianc, a forty-ninc-ycar-old divorced mother of a fifteen-year-old, confided to mc that shc had hoped her ex-husband was reaching out to her when he talked constantly about the steps he was taking to restore an old car. "It took me a long time to realize that he only wanted to talk about the car and that anyone would do as an audience. He wanted my acknowledgment and that's it—he never once asked me about my interests. I hate to say it, but our son is a chip off the old block. When he starts acting nice, asks me how my day was, or helps out more at home, I've learned to brace myself for the 'big move' just around the corner. He's gotten bold enough to give me a compliment and ask for a favor in the same sentence. If there's nothing he wants, it's the silent treatment again."

Sadly, silence can also be a form of manipulation. Some boys sense how badly important people in their lives want to connect with them. Instead of using this awareness as a signal to reach out, they use it as an opportunity for leverage. You may not be able to change your son's inclinations, but you can at least level with him about how he makes you feel when he holds out on communicating with you. After several frustrating family sessions, one parent boldly told me that on the drive home after their last session she decided she had had enough. "I told him, look, I know you don't want to talk to me, but I want you to know it really hurts me. I raised you! You're the most important thing in the world to me, and all I ever hear is 'Can I get a ride?,' 'Can I have some money?,' or 'What's for supper?' I think he finally got the message, because he's been making more of an effort. Almost every day now he remembers to at least ask me how my day was. It's a start."

When Silence Turns into Withdrawal

Parents are naturally concerned about boys who seem to withdraw into private worlds where other people are less relevant. In part, we've been conditioned to be wary of social withdrawal because of hearing so many stories about the antisocial activities of reclusive boys. Does retreating to his room behind a wall of music suggest that he's trying drugs? Are the hours on the computer healthy? There is a delicate balance between underreacting and overreacting to social withdrawal that challenges our patience and understanding.

Responding to silence or social withdrawal can be particularly difficult when parents disagree about the level of concern limited communication warrants. When do boys need space, and when should parents step in? I remember listening to the parents of a sixteen-year-old argue about his reclusiveness. "For goodness sake, Lea, he's not building bombs in the basement!" exclaimed the father. "How would you know? Would he tell you?" answered his wife. If I had to pick a side, I would guess that your son is not involved in deviant, antisocial activities if he withdraws. But I would be concerned enough to err on the side of caution, to the extent that I would gently investigate the situation until I was satisfied that the thread of communication was still intact. In some families, the withdrawal tendencies of boys don't get noticed unless there is some type of problem with academics, a behavioral issue at school, or some other type of action that moves boys into parental focus. But by then parents are in the far more difficult position of having to react to a problem than prevent one. If your son is withdrawn or shy, you'll find specific help in Chapter 5.

"Please Don't Notice My Changes"

One of our hardest jobs as parents is not to assume that we are the cause of our sons' behavior. This is not to say we shouldn't feel obligated to do anything about it. When a boy resists communication, parents might reasonably think, "Well, how else should we take this? After all, shouldn't he be comfortable talking to the people with whom he has spent the most time, the people who have loved and provided for him?" It may sound like a logical proposition, but things feel very different to boys. Ironically, for many boys the people who know them best are often those they are most concerned about shielding their deeper self from. Perhaps surprisingly, parents are uniquely qualified to make some boys feel very self-conscious. This is because you have witnessed core transformations in your son's identity, skills, and social relations, and he may have preferred those progressions to be much less obvious to the outside world, even to you.

Boys are not necessarily comfortable with the personal changes they experience over the course of childhood and adolescence. They often feel "stupid" about experiencing developmental benchmarks. And if you compliment boys about their social development, they may have mixed feelings about accepting your praise. For example, when you remark that your son has made a lot of friends in school this year, you're providing him with positive affirmation. That's a wonderful offering, but considering the intense self-consciousness of many boys, your son may not hear the compliment as you intend it. Instead, he may feel embarrassed, thinking that you are contrasting his social life now to what it was last year, when he was new to middle school and nobody talked to him. Your kind words may unintentionally have poked at an unhealed wound. Naturally, he won't be inclined to continue this conversation. Of course, I'm not suggesting you not compliment your son, but only that you be sensitive to how his life experiences might shape how he hears you.

I believe that many boys would prefer that other people see them as always having been just as they are *right now*. Presenting a steadfast personal image is one way boys assert confidence about themselves and their perspectives. Boys can also minimize their mistakes or experiences of change when they convince themselves of their clarity of purpose. A boy doesn't have to consciously reflect on the fact that he has changed his mind and image more than once and has experimented with being a different kind of person—as a normal part of growing up.

Ironically, the very process of experimentation is a source of hope for parents, a sign that boys can be flexible and have enough confidence to explore presenting a different outward image to the world. Feeling awkward about trying on new images is another point of contrast between boys and girls, particularly after about age ten. Whereas a girl typically feels comfortable trying on new clothes, spelling her name differently, and portraying different kinds of images almost as a kind of play, that process is usually uncomfortable for all but the most confident and outgoing boys by the time they reach elementary school age. Boys are socialized to feel as though they are supposed to be sure of themselves. As a consequence, trying on roles or "costumes" may be psychologically associated with a lack of confidence or some type of weakness. Although the clothes boys wear to school may be highly expressive (often including provocative words and phrases), they are expressive within the parameters of a code sanctioned by peers. Working hard to look like their peers helps boys escape the kind of attention they dread.

An important developmental step for boys involves applying learning from one situation to another. Boys in general, and adolescents in particular, tend to think in absolutes. The view that what's happening now is all-important sometimes clashes with the fear that successes can be temporary. Your role as witness of his past failures (real or perceived) may make a boy feel uncomfortable. Yet your optimism about his potential for success and acknowledgement of his accomplishments can help your son overcome these fears.

Sometimes It *Is* Just a Phase . . .

When you're confused and wonder whether some underlying emotional issue has prompted your son's retreat, it's helpful to remember that the impulse to communicate and socialize is cyclical for most people. In families where people are emotionally attuned to each other, changes in behavior can heighten everyone's anxiety. In other words, you can get much more upset about your son's sudden propensity to be silent than the situation demands. Both individually and as a family, it's normal to engage with each other and then retreat, engage and retreat. Inevitably, there will be times when boys feel less inclined to relate what they are thinking and feeling. When we as parents can be comfortable with shifting patterns of communication, our sons will be able to normalize their own experiences.

This is a tough act to pull off for many of us. Many parents these days are very involved with their kids, sometimes overinvolved, and are oversensitive to such changes in family dynamics. And the incredible stress that most of us live with can really heighten that sensitivity. But I would ask you to extend the same courtesy to your son you might show an adult family member or co-worker. Think about the signs you would look for in those people to tell you whether you should approach them or give them some space. If they were quiet with an obvious expression of distress, or if you noticed a dramatic change in their behavior or work habits, you would probably want to ask what was going on. But if they just seemed to be retreating to a more contemplative place, needing time to sort out their feelings or think through a decision, you would probably want to respect their privacy. Our sons need the same kinds of consideration. No matter how well we think we know them, we need to pay close attention to perceive the subtle signals that convey their emotional needs.

You can be helpful to your son by being patient and supportive and sending consistent signals that you're ready to hear what he has to say whenever he's ready to talk. This is often easier when you're involved with your son in activities that are less focused on emotional communication. Fathers and sons will often do their best talking when driving or fishing because those activities allow them to look someplace other than toward each other. In general, boys find it much less comfortable to communicate when they have to make eye contact with someone. Each generation of boys devises new ways of adapting to this vulnerability, such as fidgeting, hiding behind their hair, sporting a carefully placed hat, or exploiting the anonymity of sunglasses. Our eyes are a window to our minds, and as boys reach adolescence, the less you know about their minds, the more comfortable they feel. One way you can maximize your chances of communicating with your son is to simply spend more time with him. Unless there's a pressing issue, it may be most helpful to make the time task-oriented, rather than sitting down formally and saying, "Let's talk."

. . . And Sometimes Moodiness Warrants Greater Concern

There are times when boys retreat for reasons beyond their control, such as a low mood. Depression makes it harder for boys to find the words they need to connect and undermines what may already be limited motivation to reach out socially. In addition, feelings of hopelessness can lead boys to judge themselves harshly when it comes to social communication. Depressed boys focus far more on negative feedback and experiences of failure than on success. As we've seen, boys convert all kinds of feelings and self-perceptions to anger. Nine-year-old Timothy looked at me intently and said, "I don't care what anyone thinks. They're morons. They should just leave me alone. Everyone should just leave me alone."

■ ■ ■

Sometimes it's hard to differentiate between a normal period of reflection and the retreat that stems from depression. If your son is withdrawing from normal activities, is experiencing a change in appetite or sleep habits, or has become irritable or sad without apparent reason, you should have him evaluated by a professional.

"Did someone say something that hurt you?" I asked.

"I told you, I don't care."

"I'll take that as a yes," I ventured.

Rather than probe further, I suggested Tim show me his favorite Pokémon cards. "What do you like best about them?" I asked.

"They can change into something different if they want," he replied. *"This one's not stupid or scared because he can destroy other Pokémons if he needs to!"* If your son seems depressed, it is clearly in your best interest to be more active in trying to draw him out or perhaps have him seen by a professional. Judging when this level of intervention is warranted is often difficult for parents. But just as you would likely "rather be safe than sorry" when it comes to taking him to his pediatrician when he has a bad cold, it is wise to use mental health professionals if you're unsure about his emotional well-being (see Chapter 11).

He Comes By It Honestly

Some boys don't talk because their families as a whole don't communicate very much. And just as individuals have cycles of communication, so do families. Most children are quite sensitive to changes in these cycles and may unconsciously mirror those patterns in their own communication. When boys notice a communication impasse between parents, they may quickly adopt the same strategy, particularly in relating to their mothers. An uncommunicative husband may unintentionally give permission to a boy to be a communication-resistant son.

It's helpful to remember that children usually learn social behavior, including communication, from the parent of the same gender. Social communication traits tend to be modeled and passed down within families from mothers to daughters and from fathers to sons. Of course, this is not an absolute rule but generally explains why so many boys develop communication styles that echo those of their fathers. Knowing this gives fathers an extraordinary opportunity to impact the development of their sons. Yet the same biases that affect boys also shape the behavior of fathers. Fathers, like all effective teachers, must first examine how their sons learn from them. Making a significant difference in the social communication of boys requires fathers to be conscious of their own communication choices, adopting strategies that meet the relational needs of the family and the emotional needs of their sons.

Laura said she sometimes does a double take when she hears "little Bill" say something so much like what his father would say, momentarily confused about whom she's talking to! "In a way it's kind of cute, but my son can take it too far, especially if we argue. Fortunately, my husband has picked up on it and has been firm in telling our son when he's out of bounds. It's strange, but I think noticing little Bill's communication has kind of helped my husband too."

Mothers who are raising their sons alone should take these factors into account when considering male role models and mentors for them. Because boys are often unaware or unconcerned about communication deficits, they ordinarily feel no particular sense of urgency about working to change how they communicate. It is especially important to be reinforcing at those times when your son does decide to confide in you. It can take a lot of courage for him to initi-

ate communication in the first place, and you want to send an un-
equivocal message that this is important to you. In many families,
the task of reinforcing children for expressive communication too often falls on one parent's shoulders. This may not be by design, but
simply a bad habit that stems from the typical division of household
labor when children are very young. Boys need to hear that their efforts at expressive communication are valued by both parents . . .
"Right, Dad?"

A Family's Communication Is Shaped by Many Factors

When parents can look objectively at how their own patterns of
communication change as they experience different emotions, they
have a better chance of understanding how their sons have learned to
respond to their own feelings. One mother said to me, "I come from a
big Italian family, just like you see in the movies. Everybody talked
loudly and said whatever they had to say—that's just the way we
were. Yet I was attracted to my husband because he was different
from all that. I liked his calm, cool demeanor. Everything is okay except when we argue. I'm yelling and waving my arms, and he wants
to sit down and go over everything methodically. Once he even tried
to draw the problem out on paper! I'm sorry, but the way I was raised
we didn't solve family problems with diagrams and flowcharts.
What's funny is that my son changes his style to deal with us. When
he is having an issue with me, he yells back and forth with me, but if
he's got a problem with his dad, it's more like a logical debate; neither one ever gets loud. I can't wait to see what kind of girl he mar-
ries."

Other issues, such as siblings and family schedules, may also
have a significant impact on whether or not boys communicate.
When families are in constant chaos because there are many children
or many different activities, boys can feel as though what they do say
doesn't "stick." However, it probably doesn't surprise you that parents and children define effortful communication very differently.
For parents, making an honest effort to communicate means doing
whatever is necessary to get their son's attention, at least when something important has to be said or discussed. Yet for boys who would
prefer to avoid expressive or personal communication with parents
altogether, exchanges are often kept to a minimum. Even then, boys
can be clever about sandwiching important information between

more trivial matters to simultaneously distract parents and cover themselves for future reference. But it still may not prevent them from being resentful that you missed the point they were being so elliptical about!

When boys withdraw from family communication, it affects the entire family's balance, and relationships are changed. One silent person at a table can change the entire dynamic of a dinner conversation. Communication resistance can increase family tension, and the problem is compounded when parents suspect their sons may be struggling with difficult personal decisions—choices that could change their lives. Boys who need to be slowly drawn out take time and attention away from siblings. This can intensify sibling rivalry, especially when a sibling sides with the frustrations of a parent. This type of drama often characterizes the tensions between brother and sister. In addition, boys with exceptionally communicative sisters or brothers often can't stand up to the verbal sparring that takes place. As a consequence, they defensively tune their families out. Take time to step back and carefully observe your own family. Ask yourself, "Is this a hospitable environment for someone who finds personal expression difficult? Are we able to provide the time and quality of interaction our son might need to open up?"

Keeping Your Concerns in Perspective

One reason it can be hard to get through to boys is that they don't necessarily understand why parents need to know what they're thinking and feeling in the first place. Boys with a low level of social interest may not even comprehend why parents care if they talk. Remember, we all use ourselves as a reference point in trying to understand others. We tend to expect other people to think and react as we do. Yet when boys have relatively low interest in the thoughts and feelings of others, they naturally underestimate their own interest to parents. It can be very confusing to them when we express our concern about their lack of "quality" communication. Imagine if someone abducted you in the middle of the night and you awoke in another country where everyone was shouting at you in a language you didn't understand. Animated expressions and loud talk would not likely help make their language any more comprehensible.

For those of us who are communicative, it's sometimes hard to understand or accept people who are less verbally inclined. They are no less dismayed by us! Measuring our sons against some mythical, perfect image of what a boy should be is a recipe for disappointment. Even boys you may think are particularly perceptive can be devastated to realize they have fallen short of their parents' expectations. One of the saddest therapy sessions I had was with a seven-year-old who erupted in tears when his father threw his hands up in the air and exclaimed in frustration, "His brothers don't act like this, I never acted like this—what's going on with this kid?" At the time, the child had no capacity to explain what he was feeling or why he misbehaved the way he did. Yet the full weight of his father's disappointment and the impact of family comparisons was crushing. When boys can't tell us what's wrong, it may be because they can't find the words.

You're probably getting the idea that it can be difficult for a parent to know when to react to a boy who's not communicating. This is definitely a decision that requires consideration and sensitivity. Before you start worrying about whether to react to your own son's lack of communication, let me suggest that how you react to him will be the most important factor in how your concern is perceived and whether or not he responds to your concern. Find a quieter voice within yourself and trust that your expressed love and understanding will be a welcome sign that helps him across the communication divide.

Emotionally Speaking

Of the many reasons that boys resist communicating, perhaps the most telling is their discomfort in the realm of emotions. We've seen that many boys are more comfortable working with tangible things and facts than making sense of feelings. You've met boys whose confusion about what they're feeling only encourages them to avoid the realm of emotions because they feel at sea there. And we've talked about boys who end up disserving themselves by relying on anger as their default because it's the only emotion they know how to express. But boys' uneasiness with emotion has even deeper roots and far-reaching implications. Emotional illiteracy threatens to unravel the potential of so many otherwise promising young men. And your understanding of this phenomenon is at the heart of your ability to make a critical difference in your son's life.

FOUR

Without Words for Emotion

■ ■ ■

One of the great challenges of our generation is to get out of our own heads to make time and space for others. By making time and space, we clear a path to the very heart of ourselves, enabling the closeness that makes life fulfilling. All of us, and perhaps especially parents, devote considerable energy and attention to the myriad responsibilities of daily life. For most people, time and space are at a premium, dimensions of life that can feel like scarce commodities. We work on one project while attending to another in the background, all the while planning what the next step will be— what we will *do* next. Yet one of the greatest gifts we can offer another person is the gift of time and attention. Through our thoughtful attention and receptivity to others we invite people to become known to us. When we are in this place, we are far removed from distraction, anxiety, and self-absorption. We are open, aware, and listening; our attention can move beyond the boundaries of our own self-interests; our words will reflect what we hear deeply. This is the spirit of empathy, and it is communication that brings it to life.

Empathy is the ability to see through the eyes of others, to feel what others feel. It's more than sympathy—feeling sorry for someone—which at times may be important but still leaves a chasm between us and others. With empathy we momentarily subordinate our own views or opinions for the sake of *feeling* how something is experienced by someone else. Doing this closes the gap between us and others and leads us to act in accordance with our social conscience. Boys who have developed the ability to feel empathy are able to form closer relationships with others and are more likely to allow others to

79

enter their own psychological space. The ability to view the world from someone else's perspective is a great antidote to self-absorption because it draws one into the realm of other people.

We all function in various types of groups—couples, families, schools, teams, communities, and workplaces, among others—and our sons are no exception. Participating to our full potential in these groups means fulfilling our longing to be understood and to give of ourselves to others. If our sons are to function successfully and happily in all these arenas, they will need to make empathy an integral part of their lives, bringing it to life through words and deeds.

Empathy provides the energy and motivation to cross the communication divide. Developing a vocabulary of emotions is a primary way boys both express empathy and hone it—this is the principle of behavioral bidirectionality in action. Our sons have at least some natural instinct for empathy, but we need to cultivate it.

Are We Unwittingly Anti-Empathy?

We want our sons to be bright, athletic, and well behaved, but we rarely focus on their empathy, even though it's an important aspect of their social development. Communities everywhere hold certain expectations about what kinds of academic or team performance are desirable; parents everywhere discuss these topics intensely. But how often do we talk about—even think about—how our sons should understand and treat others? I'd venture to say that it's easier for more fathers, standing on the sidelines, to admonish their sons to "kick butt" than to "play fair." What about the mom who reserves her tutelage in being "nice," and the social insight it requires, for her daughters? Often, we limit our training of boys to managing their behavior ("don't hit"), without taking the next step of exploring the motivations behind bad behavior, discussing better alternatives for action, and building empathy by considering the impact on the victim ("How do you think Andrew felt when you took his toy away?").

Do We Teach Boys That Winning Is Everything?

Unfortunately, many of us have accepted this situation as natural for boys. We may even encourage a lack of empathy in boys in a misguided attempt at making them "stronger" or to express our own underlying aggression. It's easy to find ourselves living vicariously through our sons' competitive exploits. As a result we may unconsciously reinforce conquest as life's greatest virtue. Believe me, though, boys don't need any help in getting this message. They are surrounded by images that dramatize the merits of being victorious, and they are hardwired to keep these images in the forefront of their minds. As parents, we have to work hard not to become unwitting collaborators in validating the dominant social message to be competitive, to the exclusion of all other ways of relating to others. We should not ask our sons to be symbols or surrogates of our own achievement. They will be unfairly weighed down by this burden or, alternatively, become emotionally lopsided in their quest to win at all costs.

Raising Lone Rangers

If we're not discouraging empathy by overemphasizing the value of conquests, we're contributing to unempathic behavior by lionizing the well-adjusted loner. That loners are so healthy is a myth that pervades popular entertainment and is an outright denial of men's emotional needs. We deeply romanticize males whose individuality is too strong to be socialized. Their unwillingness to adopt social conventions is often depicted as a kind of iconoclastic heroism. Incredibly, we are shocked when boys take these ideas seriously, becoming aggressive with other boys in the backyard, acting in open defiance of

▪ ▪ ▪

Doesn't Empathy Come Naturally?

Many believe the germ is there in all of us. But we're often unaware of how easy it is to stunt its growth. Here are some of the ways we unwittingly thwart our sons' empathy:

- Equating expressions of emotion or empathy with weakness—sometimes in the name of keeping our sons safe in a "hard world"
- Egging them on to act out our own underlying aggression
- Perpetuating negative stereotypes of "sensitive" men and supporting the myth of the iconoclastic hero
- Consistently stressing action to the neglect of reflection

parents, even taking a gun to school to enforce their own version of right and wrong.

It *is* a hard world, without a doubt. So hard that at times probably all of us harbor a secret wish to cast aside the burden of social expectations—the need to understand other people—difficult in-laws, impossible co-workers, aggravating neighbors, faceless bureaucrats who "have no record of our payment" or reject our insurance claims—and how to "deal" with them. The disappointments and frustrations of life can make defying the dehumanizing aspects of social conformity seem like a pretty romantic notion. But we have to ask ourselves if turning our backs on the complexity and social demands of our world is a realistic or appropriate model for males in the twenty-first century. As adults, where will our sons find the motivation to work on a difficult marriage or relate to their own children? Who will inspire them to be of service to others? How will they know when a compromise is the greatest victory?

Larger Than Life or Grandiose?

Of course, it's not just the messages that we give our sons—intentionally or unintentionally—that foster or discourage empathy. Stereotypes that surround us make it difficult for boys to be comfortable with sensitively expressed emotion, partly because prevalent images of manhood trickle down to the youngest males. Even the most emotionally sophisticated adults often react with distaste to men who freely express all kinds of emotion, with the possible exception of the "outraged hero." Look at the typical "action" film or other movie marketed to the male audience; you'll notice a lot of male heroes who get really, really mad. Battling various forms of humiliation and indignity (the universal male fears), the hero works to assert his might, rationalizing that violence is necessary to the pursuit of justice. The film may be laced with occasional references to needing others, perhaps for sex or medical care, but mostly what the hero needs is admirers. And so our sons are repeatedly exposed to the perverse idea that heroism and grandiosity are one and the same and that, among powerful men, action diminishes the need for words.

Although most of us can differentiate between fantasy entertainment and reality, this is something we should think about, because clichés do tell us something about what's going on in our minds. If we look at successful leaders in public life—teachers, politicians, doctors, CEOs, even the actors who *portray* the angry men in films—we see that these are generally men who are greatly appreciated for their ability to relate and communicate. I believe most parents want their sons to acknowledge such role models. Unfortunately, there are few compelling movies or songs about such men, and most adolescent boys have limited patience for public television! We have a right to ask the extraordinary talent found among the major mediums of television, film, and music to use their creativity to benefit, rather than exploit, the social and emotional needs of youth. As parents, we have the responsibility to seek and support media that doesn't compromise aesthetics *or* values—they needn't be mutually exclusive. Where are the reality shows that show us how to live an honorable life? Please vote with your dollars. Support high-quality children's media with your purchases and recommendations to other parents; and don't spend your hard-earned wages on entertainment that exploits the vulnerability of boys with messages of triumph through aggression—they're simply too young to understand that these ideas are far more about fantasy than healthy life skills.

Learning the Language of Emotions

You probably wouldn't be reading this book if you didn't agree that boys should learn to express their thoughts and feelings and empathize with those of others. But holding this belief doesn't tell any of us *how* to instill empathy in our sons—especially if we're worried about the risk of making them "oversensitive" or vulnerable to the attacks of *less* empathetic boys.

I remember being in the supermarket and noticing a young child crying because one of his toy cars had been accidentally crushed by a shopping cart. Having been in a similar situation with my own son, I offered his father what I thought was a smile of reassurance and identification. Unfortunately, my acknowledgment seemed to heighten his self-consciousness, as he quickly averted his eyes and snapped at his son, "Stop it, you're acting like a baby."

This father's reaction reflects one of our society's unspoken rules about male emotion: Crying is for babies. Although we're not surprised when babies cry to communicate their basic needs, we often expect slightly older boys to suppress that instinct. Maybe you've found yourself feeling some discomfort with boys who cry past the age of three or four, especially in public. Sometimes we get embarrassed, like the father in the grocery store, and act as though we want even our youngest sons to avoid expressing their feelings at all. But usually it's not that we want them to shut down; rather, that we expect them to start using words instead of tears to convey their feelings.

The trouble is, we don't provide boys with a basic vocabulary for emotional literacy. We often assume they will just magically "get it." Unconsciously, we may show our daughters how to express their feelings more thoroughly, while it is our sons who may need the most direct coaching.

> ■ ■ ■
>
> When your son cries, notice what may be causing his distress and help articulate it for him: "Are you frustrated that your brother wins more than you?" or "Sometimes it's hard to feel patient when you're waiting for Mom to help you, isn't it?" Boys are inventive. Give them the tools they need to do a job, in this case specific words, and they will make industrious, creative use of them. The right tools make all the difference.

Empathy requires a specific kind of language—a language of emotions. Without a working vocabulary for emotions, we are limited in our capacity both to express and to comprehend emotional states. Perhaps you can remember certain key times in your life when your emotional sensitivity and your ability to verbalize that sensitivity were highly valuable. Maybe you were able to say just the right words to comfort a grieving friend or were able to head off a serious confrontation with someone who was angry by "talking him down." For boys, the expression of sensitivity often occurs in a somewhat roundabout manner. This is because most boys are not inclined to openly interpret or declare feelings. That does not mean, however, that they are incapable of sensing emotions or responding supportively.

Not long ago, I was leading a group I call Mighty Good Kids™ for second- and third-grade boys. The purpose of the group was for the boys to develop better social skills. We were huddled in my office with kids crowded on sofas, sitting on the floor, and twirling in my desk chair. One seven-year-old boy, Jordan, resisted joining in our group activity, which was to draw pictures of good and bad ways to handle anger. He stood near the door on the periphery of the group with a hesitant expression and body language that conveyed his fear and distrust of others. Jordan wasn't responding to cajoling and encouragement to join us. I tried some different approaches, changing the tone of my voice and my own facial expression, in search of a combination that would help him join in. Still, he would not budge. Years ago, I probably would have taken Jordan outside and pleaded with him to sit down and join the group. That's because I used to have the faulty impression that *leading* a group meant *controlling* the group. Since then I've come to appreciate the extraordinarily strong will of boys to do things in ways that reflect their own logic about how problems should be solved.

As the situation unfolded, it became apparent that Jordan's resistance provided the boys with a good problem-solving opportunity, and so I posed a question to the group. Did anyone have any ideas about how we could get Jordan to join us? Most of the kids responded with suggestions of various kinds of rewards: games, candy, or premium seating (twirling chair). One typically shy boy, Tyler, suggested we could "buddy up" so that everyone would have a partner, including Jordan. Tyler also suggested that buddies sit next to each other so they could share markers. Most of the boys agreed this was a good idea, and so we began a discussion of how buddies would be chosen. Again, Tyler spoke up, suggesting that Jordan should pick his buddy.

Throughout this process I was watching Jordan closely and was struck by his awareness of the group's concern about him. His facial expression changed from one of distrust to a sheepish grin. He had obviously had some significant doubt about whether the boys would accept him and how he would fit in—figuratively and literally. Tyler's leadership in breaking through this doubt had paved the way for Jordan to become part of the group. As you might imagine, I felt very proud of Tyler for his sensitivity to Jordan and his ability to apply that sensitivity through active problem solving. Although he never identified a particular feeling, Tyler's suggestions were, emotionally speaking, quite sophisticated. Even while using a goal-oriented, "male" way of communicating, through his suggestions he demonstrated that he understood (empathized with) what Jordan was feeling. In essence, Tyler had offered ideas that made it easier for Jordan to save face and feel secure.

We Are What We Say

No doubt you've heard the expression "We are what we do." Well, as I visit schools, work with families, and meet with boys in therapy, I am continually struck by how much what boys do comes down to what they say, at least as far as fortifying their self-concept—the way they see and understand themselves—is concerned. In essence, *the language boys use and how they communicate play a formative role in shaping their identity and character.* When they develop the skills of empathic communication, they grow into men who move with ease and agility in the social world. They are confident and comfortable with themselves and compassionate toward others. Again, this is the very essence of the bi-directional relationship between communication and a boy's understanding of himself. Your son's words are shaping who he will become.

There are two primary ways this shaping process takes place. First, we are all witnesses to our own behavior. We learn about ourselves from the way in which we do particular things. For instance, if a boy is taught a code of politeness at an early age, his behavior is likely to reflect that learning as he gets older. Almost unconsciously, he simply acts that way because it's familiar and habitual. As the watchful, self-reflective part of his mind observes himself doing and saying polite things, an important self-awareness takes root: "I am a polite person." Through this process an important aspect of his self-concept is solidified. Politeness graduates from being merely a reflexive habit to being a behavior driven by a desire to act in accordance with his beliefs about himself. Behaviors build the core of our beings.

This is a powerful process because the self-concept we build from thoughtful, constructive behavior is like a microchip that tells our mind how to think, feel, and act in a variety of situations. Self-concepts that are developed in childhood or adolescence also tend to endure into adulthood and may be tough to change—ask any therapist, or consider your own efforts to change your most fundamental beliefs about who you are. This is why it's so important to contribute to shaping our sons' healthy self-concepts or self-beliefs early in life. These strongly held self-beliefs feel more like "truths" than beliefs and will guide our sons' development for years to come. For example, if your son is taught to be considerate of the elderly and infirm ("We give up our seats on the bus for someone who can't stand easily"), he grows up subscribing to the belief that "I am a kind person." This personal trait translates to "I am a caring husband, a nurturing father, an appreciative boss" as he grows older.

The second way shaping occurs is through the feedback boys receive about their actions and choices. We all receive a steady stream of verbal and nonverbal communication in response to our actions. In other words, we notice the reactions we get in response to our behavior. This stream of information has a cumulative effect in shaping how we think about ourselves. So, if a boy is consistently polite, he is likely to receive verbal feedback positively acknowledging that behavior—and reinforcing his self-concept as a polite individual. Reinforcement is effective because it feels good to be told we're doing something well.

The cause and effect of behavioral shaping may sound simple, but the net effect is powerful: to your son, when you comment on his actions you are using *your* words to express your innermost thoughts and feelings about him. Sometimes, your love and positive regard is so much a "given" that it's easy to forget to articulate those feelings when you have them toward your son. Yet when you remember to notice his better traits and actions aloud, you not only help form your son's positive conception of himself, but affirm your appreciation of him—a strong motivator toward further social development. It's easy to see, then, that as parents we have a significant responsibility to teach and reinforce socially positive behavior. We will best meet the demands of that responsibility if we recognize that our efforts can dramatically improve the emotional life of boys, now and in the future.

You might take small verbal gestures such as "please" or "it's nice to see you" for granted, yet they

> ■ ■ ■
>
> A boy's perspective of himself, sometimes called his *self-concept*, grows from witnessing his own behavior and is reinforced by the responses of others to his actions. Once developed, such self-concepts are very difficult to change. How does your son think about himself? What behaviors (including communication) contribute to his beliefs?

are the incremental steps that lead to social interest. In fact, the social conscience of boys is built on these microskills of social communication. If your son uses simple social expressions in a way that strikes you as superficial or unfelt, ask yourself if you've forgotten to emphasize the sentiments, such as consideration for others, that should underlie those words.

The simple phrases we use, such as "please" and "thank you," are verbal acknowledgments of the importance of others. When we speak in a courteous way, we indicate interest in others, respect for their importance, and care for their feelings. Because of this, such words are powerful. We loan prized possessions, grant forgiveness, attend amateur recitals, and give out raises all for hearing the word *please*; we write large donor checks, drive friends to the airport, and knock ourselves out on the job, asking only "thanks" in return. If you're in a grocery line and someone says, "Excuse me, I'm sorry to bother you, but would you please let me go ahead with just this one thing?—I wouldn't ask, but I'm really late for an appointment," chances are you'll let that person cut in, even if it inconveniences you. Imagine if the same person said, "I need to go first—I'm late. I only have one thing." While factually correct and to the point, this self-absorbed request is more likely to be denied or resented because it doesn't acknowledge the other person's feelings. Polite words grease the wheels of a society in which we all must shift and accommodate the needs and desires of many people. Polite words acknowledge the selflessness required to participate in communal society and reflect others' appreciation of our individuality within this group structure. When we show our sons how to be thoughtful in their remarks to others—"I'm glad you're driving me because you always tell such funny stories along the way"—rather than a perfunctory "Thanks for the ride," we not only teach them how to like others, but increase their own chances of being well regarded.

Getting through Barbed Wire

Early exposure to the *hows* and *whys* of social communication skills is particularly important for boys who may have marginal self-confidence. Through effective communication they can experience a sense of competence and mastery complementary to their need for confidence. When boys anticipate failure, they inevitably opt for avoidance because deep down inside a voice is telling them to avoid embarrassment and humiliation at all costs, even if that means social withdrawal. Boys are experts at shutting down and making you feel like an intruder in their personal lives. Sometimes I joke with kids that they have to take down their "no trespassing" sign when they come into my office! Some boys grin and get the point, but others find even the slightest reference to their feelings embarrassing, becoming even more adamant about controlling any expression of emotion. Remember, most boys struggle with showing signs of vulnerability or what they perceive to be weakness. The messages we send our sons are potent, and the energy they expend trying to live up to our expectations represents a significant commitment of their psychological resources. Given such an investment, shouldn't we give our sons a better script to work with?

Several years ago I was counseling a former military officer turned executive. Our sessions focused on how he could more effectively motivate his subordinates. James was intense, organized, and matter-of-fact. He could process complex information very quickly and held high standards for his employees and himself. As with many high achievers, it took little more than a suggestion for him to make exponential improvements in the way he conducted business.

James also held very high standards for his son and was more than a little frustrated that his son did not share his enthusiasm for a well-managed life. Gradually, our sessions shifted to conversation about James's concern for James Jr. He remarked, "You know, I don't know if there is a real problem; certainly there's nothing diagnosable. It's something I can't put my finger on. My son is twelve, he's big for his age, he's in kind of an awkward stage. He's not in any trouble and he isn't a bad student, but sometimes I'm not sure I know who he is anymore." He paused. "Maybe you should talk to him," James suggested. I agreed to do that.

At twelve years old, James Jr. was almost six feet tall. He wore big baggy jeans that sagged halfway down his rear end and a gray sweatshirt in which he kept his hands tucked. He shuffled across my office in sneakers without laces and slumped in the far corner of the sofa, clearly expressing his feelings about having to talk to me. His leg rocked back and forth impatiently. As I introduced myself I couldn't help thinking what a striking contrast there was between father and son.

We went through the usual initial questions, and James Jr. obliged with, variously, "I don't know," "I don't really care," "No," "Nothing," "Not really," and finally snarled, "Do I have to be here?"

Defensive boys like James Jr. defy anyone who tries to reach them. They hide behind a wall of indifference, and when the wall threatens to crumble, they resort to the one overused emotion they know—anger. When in doubt about what to say or how to respond, they push the anger button, hoping to intimidate and shut down any attempt to be close to them. Indifference is intended to signal that they know themselves and their minds well enough not to need anyone else. These boys deceive themselves into thinking that others will interpret their anger as power and self-confidence.

Despite his size, and willingness to be surly, I suspected that James Jr. wasn't as indifferent as he was pretending to be. His "street" attire had been assembled carefully to express rebellion. Sometimes boys who are large for their age are expected to be tough and are either challenged by other boys trying to make their mark or "invited," despite their age, to follow a pack of older kids. The look and attitude are part of the camouflage needed to blend in. The clothes could also have been a way of rebelling against his father, a fastidious dresser who undoubtedly would disapprove of his son's apparel choices. As I was mulling this over, I asked James Jr. if he ever got into fights in school.

"Huh?" he asked, looking surprised. "Me?"

"Yeah, you," I replied. "Ever get into it with anyone?"

James Jr. conveyed the basics of his beliefs on the subject. "I don't look for trouble, but I'm not afraid of anyone either. I can handle myself all right."

"So you've handled yourself? What did you do?" I asked.

"What do you mean?" he replied.

"Have you ever hit anyone? Made a fist?"

"Well, I don't have to really. People know not to mess with me." He leaned back and shrugged, crossing his arms. "There's kids at my school who—well, put it this way—I'm glad I'm not them." I was struck by how much more verbal James Jr. had become as the topic had shifted to something in which he clearly had an emotional investment. Talking about tension with other boys in school was the "frequency" on which James Jr. was ready to be heard. As we talked, he seemed to connect strongly with the topic, and the more questions I asked, the more excitedly he would relate his observations of what was going on between other students in school. He began to make sweeping statements: "In this world you have to stand up for yourself," "There are winners and losers," "Never let nobody see your fear," and "It's a hard world." For the first time, I could begin to hear the commonalities between father and son. These statements were an adapted version of the work ethic of his father, who frequently talked about remaining tough and unemotional when it came to business.

Later, when I met with his father, we discussed the themes of the conversation. I repeated the phrases that James Jr. had used with me, as his father, smiling and slightly embarrassed, put his head in his hands. "Talk about taking things out of context!" he said. "I spoke with him a lot about the merger. Everyone was panicked, and my staff was taking cues from me. As a leader, I had to stand tough. At times, I had to be assertive; sometimes I bluffed, even when I was worried we'd all be out of work. But he missed the point. The reason I did these things was to motivate people, get the best from them, develop their skills and keep them employed. They wouldn't follow me anywhere if there wasn't mutual trust and respect." Once again, I made some supportive suggestions to James, including spending time talking with his son about the things that mattered most to James Jr. As usual, he got the message quickly. After periodic check-ins for a few months, I didn't hear back from him. But a half year later I received a photo of James and James Jr. in the mail. They had an arm around each other's shoulders, smiling and holding up some striped bass, caught on a fishing trip. In his rapid scrawl, James had written, "Things are going well, though it's a 'hard world' for fish." The expressions of father and son suggested to me that the barbed wire had come down.

As parents, when we use the language and topics that speak to our sons' emotional realities, we are meeting them in a place where they have a reasonably good chance of responding to us. Finding the right frequency comes from both instinct (derived from spending enough time with our boys to really know them) and inquiry. The boys may try to turn us away, but usually that is because our approach is not hitting the mark. Even when we think our sons are drifting, they carry within them parts of us. Our language and ways of communicating inevitably become part of the way our sons think. Our job is not to prevent this phenomenon, but to be conscious that it is happening and nurture its healthy development. After all, by paying attention to what we pass on to our sons, we're helping them create a mental roadmap to effective social communication.

Making Maps for Social Communication

On an interpersonal level, empathy can be understood as a kind of expressed concern for others. On a cognitive or thinking level, empathy is composed of a series of maps that psychologists call *schemas*. These maps or schemas are the lenses through which a boy sees himself and his social world. Schemas become his guideposts, his reference points; the perspectives he returns to over and over to make sense out of various situations. We all develop our mental maps through experience and by learning. Learning how to think empathically includes watching others and encoding (remembering) ideas of appropriate behavior and communication in specific contexts. This process underscores why parental example is extremely important. Children are constantly watching and listening for clues to how to act. Over time, these clues become defined and organized as a kind of mental handbook for the range of options available for how to act or communicate.

Imagine a five-year-old boy watching his father at the funeral of his aunt. It is the first time this boy has seen such an effusive expression of emotion from his father, and it makes the child uneasy. He doesn't know how to react. At age five he's not sure what he is supposed to feel and is somewhat overwhelmed by the situation. The number of people crying further confuses him about why people cry. It may be the first time in his life that he experiences crying as an accepted, "normal" behavior. He notices that although people are crying, they aren't mad at each other. Instead, they often touch hands and hug. His ears are wide awake too—people are saying kind things to each other and nice things about his aunt. Although he doesn't entirely understand what's going on, he can guess that something important has brought these people together and that it's okay for people to show these feelings.

As the service ends, the child watches how his father embraces others who are in attendance. He listens to how his father thanks people for coming and how his father tells people "how much she loved you." He sees the impact of his father's words and hears the genuine tone in his father's voice. As a result, this very young boy develops a *schema* for how people, including his father, cope with situations in which strong, sad emotions are involved. He sees his father expressing emotion without anxiety or embarrassment and observes that his father seems to feel somewhat relieved to be around other family members. The child's schema for this event will include learning that sometimes the strong expression of emotion is a good thing and that by expressing emotion even grown men can feel better.

In contrast to this example, some boys grow up in families where the expression of emotion is not encouraged and is even overtly censored. *Encouraging emotional repression lays down a powerful and potentially destructive schema in boys.* How many times have you heard (or said), "Big boys don't cry" or more subtle cues like "Pull yourself together." These comments often reflect a family's or individual parent's level of discomfort with emotion—the belief that emotional expression is not manly or polite. Even worse is the erroneous and dangerous conviction that if we repress unpleasant emotions they will go away. Instead, they become more entrenched, and it is only a matter of time before those feelings will demand to be heard.

Help Him Find the Words He Needs to Feel

For many years psychologists have been aware that articulating and expressing emotions is a major hurdle for some people. Psychologists have named this syndrome *alexithymia,* which translates from Latin into "without words for emotion," and it's is no coincidence that therapists are intimately acquainted with the syndrome. It can cause major problems in marriage, within families, and at the workplace. A very high percentage of people struggling with this type of expressive hurdle are men. Often, these men find therapy to be a difficult and alien experience—probably because it requires them to do the very thing they find most challenging.

Because boys are rarely without the capacity to express at least one major emotion—anger—it seems to me that a better description of the syndrome is *dyslexithymia,* or *"inadequate* words for emotion." Just as someone with dyslexia has trouble reading, someone with dyslexithymia has trouble feeling and expressing. Dyslexithymia can be a subtle disability, because our society is not in the habit of consciously screening for poor emotional communication. Instead, we have attributed this tendency to stereotypical male characteristics such as being "strong and silent." Sometimes we mask the problem by directing our appraisal of males elsewhere—"he's good with his hands" or "he's rough around the edges, but his heart's in the right place."

■ ■ ■

Dyslexithymia, or "inadequate words for emotion," is more than just psychological jargon. This common social disability has potentially harmful effects on the mind and body. The suppression of emotions has been linked with hormonal changes, for example, that disable critical immune system functions. Sadly, when males are unable to articulate their feelings, they may be at greater risk for poor health.

Helping our sons access the words they need to make themselves and their emotions known is serious business. Yet we can make it a part of daily family life, such as discussing a scene from a television show where emotions were well articulated. Clever parents can subtly integrate their comments within normal conversation to avoid making this feel like a "lesson." Relate the situation to your own child's life! Be on the lookout for teaching opportunities. Don't be afraid to stop and provide verbal commentary for an interaction you come across in the supermarket, on the playground, or at a religious service. One of the most frequent recommendations I make to parents of boys I have evaluated for social problems is to learn to narrate the nuances of social interaction, using words and phrases that expand and deepen a boy's insight. This might involve doing a play-by-play analysis of other kids playing or arguing, or it might involve discreet "people watching" at the mall, trying to guess other people's moods.

Suppose you're sitting in the food court at a mall with your young son. Several tables away, you see a mother with a son and daughter. As they go to take their seats, the younger daughter takes the chair the son had obviously intended to sit on. After they are seated, the boy pulls some food away from his sister, who begins to fuss. The mother reprimands

■ ■ ■

It's Never Too Early . . .

You can begin to develop your son's emotional literacy at birth. Every interaction presents an opportunity to "turn on" the neural pathways for reciprocal communication. By the time your son can distinguish different kinds of vehicles or name the colors, he's old enough to start noticing and identifying feelings. If you model these kinds of observations, and coach them in your son, he will infer that this is an important type of self-awareness and in most cases will try to win your approval by showing you "I can do it."

both children and sets some cookies out of their reach across the table. Later, the mother lets the children pick cookies, and the sister offers one to her brother. A good opportunity has been presented to explore social behavior with your son. Why did the boy take his sister's food away? Suggest that he might be angry at his sister because she sat where he wanted to sit or that he's frustrated that his mother did not make his sister move. Mention that the sister is younger and may just be learning how to share, and ask him if he knows other small children who have trouble sharing and why that might be. Ask why the mother scolded them and set the cookies away from them. See if he notices that the sister was trying to be friendly to her brother by offering him a cookie and suggest that she might feel bad for taking his seat. Ask your son if the boy might also feel bad about taking his sister's food. Does he think the mother is proud of her children when they're getting along?

As your son grows in emotional literacy, he'll be able to move from simple descriptions such as *mad, sad, happy* to words that pinpoint emotions much more subtly—*frustrated, embarrassed, excited, showing-off, pleased*, and so forth. Start at a level that he's comfortable with and expand from there. Again, this can happen within the course of normal conversation, so it doesn't have to feel like "a teaching moment" to your son. He'll just learn that you are aware of other people's feelings and motivations and begin developing those valuable life skills himself. The younger you start with him, the better. If a toddler can identify several different kinds of construction trucks or name the colors, he's old enough to start noticing and categorizing feelings in himself and others.

If you haven't begun this kind of dialogue with your son, start today, or if he's reluctant to take part, simply continue trying. We cannot hope to construct the emotional architecture of our children in a week, month, or year. Yet in most cases we can begin to see at least some benefit almost immediately. Whether or not our sons fully integrate what they learn from us has a lot to do with how well we reinforce that learning through positive acknowledgment. Remember, you are the front line in the battle for your own child's emotional literacy. Boys will detect the fervor with which you wage that battle and will use your zeal as a gauge for the importance of the message.

What if you see that barbed wire fence go up again? When faced with the passionate belief of an adult, a favorite tactic of many boys is to be smug and indifferent. They want you to see that they're unmoved by your belief because they're deeply invested in being seen as sure of themselves and at least as smart as you are. I would speculate that there isn't an adult on the planet who hasn't been frustrated in trying to teach something to an overconfident, occasionally cocky boy. Yet being an effective teacher means you stay focused on what you're trying to teach and avoid getting drawn into a power struggle over who knows most. This is especially important for fathers, who sometimes get baited into a competition for control. Don't forget that even when you think your words are falling on deaf ears, your convictions and passion are messages in themselves. Convictions communicate that it's okay to care deeply about something, to express that emotion, and to have that emotion seen by others. Constructive, well-directed emotion is the rocket fuel of effective parenting. Still, it's no guarantee of a smooth flight. Attempting to get a boy to shape his behavior in accordance with parental expectations may lead to indignation and occasional conflict, but failing to care enough to convey parental beliefs and expectations is much worse—leading boys to loneliness, confusion, and self-doubt.

Let me share a favorite passage from a novel called *A Place on Earth* by Wendell Berry. In it, a father is describing how his son, Virgil, helped build a barn with his uncle Ernest.

> I reinforced the loft and put on a new roof when Virgil was thirteen or fourteen years old. It was about the first man's work he ever did. I sent him over here with Ernest and they did it together. It would worry me to death trying to get any work out of him then, but he'd work for Ernest. I saw how that was and remembered how it was with me. Mighty hard to get a boy to come to it right under his daddy's hand. . . .
>
> By the time a boy gets big enough to work, his daddy's already been his boss for a long time, and not always an easy one. They've already pretty well tested each other, and know each other's weaknesses and flaws. There are a lot of old irritations all ready-made. And then a man teaching his own boy gets misled by pride. What he does wrong looks like your failure as much as it is his, and so you don't correct or punish for his sake, but yours. The way around it—or the way my daddy took with me and I took with Virgil—is to let him work with somebody older than he is, like Ernest, that you know he admires.

There is wonderful wisdom about the dynamics between fathers and sons in that passage, and also a helpful suggestion. A wise parent not only conveys his own expectations, but also encourages his son to learn from, and develop a sense of mastery from, others. Sometimes the best way to get your message through is to find the right messenger.

Encourage Expression

Scientists involved in the study of language acquisition have developed detailed theories about the structural components of language. They have also theorized how a child's brain develops the "tools" needed to construct meaningful communication. Despite these developments, the importance of *emotion in language* has received relatively little attention. As a result, the link between language and emotions has not been fully understood. The notable linguist Lois Bloom points out that the emphasis on the "instrumental" dimension of language—how language helps children get things done—is perhaps less important than how language helps us express those aspects of human experience whose meaning is distilled in potent, evocative words. Need an example? Think of some of the most powerful words we know: *love, hate, faith, evil.* Grasping the meaning of evoca-

▪ ▪ ▪

We can use words in different ways:

- Goal-directed, instrumental speech that is problem solving and focused on achieving a particular task or obtaining specific facts: "Uncle Bob invited me to visit him next August. There's a boat show in his town next September, so I'd like to go then instead. I'll call and ask if I can come then so I can see the show, and also ask if he finished fencing his yard. If he has, maybe I can take my dog with me so that I don't have to pay to have her boarded."

- Process-oriented speech, which is evocative, expressive, and reflective and can convey the complexity of ideas and feelings: "Del's theatrical. When she flares up, she gets carried away on a wave of emotion and there's a part of her that really enjoys flying out of control—that's when she says really wild, hurtful things. But eventually she rides the wave back to shore and feels all washed out and terribly ashamed of the spectacle she made of herself. The remorse doesn't last, though, because she likes hitting that crescendo."

tive and expressive words empowers a person to use them in specific ways to convey the complexity of ideas or feelings.

Verbally disinclined boys often find it hard to shift from problem-solving language to more expressive speech. Without such speech, social skills such as self-reflection and interpersonal aware-ness become much more difficult to achieve. Imagine that you go out to buy a special red coat and find that the store is out of the adver-tised special. Clerk #1 tells you, "We're out of the red coats. We only have black and orange coats left. You can go to the service desk at the back of the store and fill out a raincheck form." Clerk #2 exclaims, "Oh, that's too bad—you came all the way down here and those were nice coats! I hope we get a red one in for you. Why don't you get a raincheck from the service desk back there? We'll be sure to call you if we get one in." The facts of the situation remain the same, but the speech of the two clerks conveys very different information to the shopper.

Because males tend to be problem solvers by nature, it makes sense that their language would typically be goal directed, having a strong instrumental orientation. However, an orientation toward problem solving and "cause and effect" type thinking can oppose em-pathy. That's because empathic communication is not so much *goal directed* as *process oriented*. This is precisely the kind of communication that boys with low verbal sensitivity find difficult and unnatural. Verbally disinclined boys often find it hard to shift their thinking from how to resolve a problem to more introspective processes such as self-reflection and interpersonal awareness. It's as if you got fired from your job and focused only on where to get a new one, rather than taking some time to consider how your behavior and relations on the job may have contributed to your being fired! Without that analysis, your problem solving occurs on a superficial level only. This sometimes happens with boys who lose a lot of friends, who then focus on finding new buddies without noticing that it was their behavior—bossiness, for example—that drove the others away. I am not advocating that boys be taught to brood or emote all the time, but I do believe boys need to be able to turn their attention inward when it is in their best interest to do so.

Feeling and expressing emotions is an integral part of the human experience, from the very first moments of life. Males have and need just as many emotions as females, and pretending they don't neither defuses them nor lessens their impact on our lives. What pretending to be emotion-free *can* do is lower our resistance to disease. It can also prevent the natural course of emotional states like grief, leaving us unable to adapt to and move on following the inevitable losses in our lives. Perhaps one of the most important things we teach our sons is that it's okay to feel whatever you feel, but "let me show you how to express those feelings in a way that actually helps you feel better." The value of this approach is difficult to overstate because it underscores that individual feelings are neither good nor bad; it's how we use them that gives them value and shapes how we will be perceived by others.

Perhaps it is unintentional, but implicit in the activities we recommend for boys is the suggestion that action and achievement—in contrast to process, reflection, and awareness—are preferred states of being. There is a subtle irony in a society that encourages men to be athletic yet at the same time fosters the type of emotional repression linked to physical disease. It reminds me of my former neighbor, who tried to stay in shape by running with his Doberman. He expended so much energy berating the dog and getting mad at pedestrians obstructing his way that I suspect his effort was misplaced; a course in anger management might have been a better cure for his heart than his daily "exercise" in frustration.

Missing the Point of the Story—Including His Own

In my work with children, I often administer a projective test that requires the child to imagine and verbalize stories about a series of picture cards with ambiguous meanings. The cards depict people with strong emotions, sometimes in conflict with others. This is a great test for assessing verbal sophistication as well as emotional perception. What is most important to me is to find out whether a boy has learned to apply words to observations in such a way that he can extract meaning from his experience of the world.

When taking this test, boys of few words have a tendency to keep their statements short and concrete. Their stories are primarily descriptive of the most obvious elements of a picture. Lee, an eleven-year-old with dyslexia, as well as social skills problems such as awkwardness and withdrawal that are frequently associated with that syndrome, described a picture of a woman crying in her hands while a man walks out a door behind her this way: "She's rubbing her face.

He has to go out. Maybe he has to go to the store." Curt, a six-year-old boy whose speech is sparse and soft, describes a picture of expressive bears engaged in a tug-of-war as "They're holding a rope. They want to get it. One bear could get wet." Compare his response to the answer a five-year-old girl gave me as she pointed out the figures: "These bears are at a party, and they want to play tug-of-war because they got bored. There are mostly girls on that side, but those ones are boys. On the other side here are all sisters and their little brothers. This one's the boss because she really wants her team to win. But that one is getting mad because the one behind him didn't pull hard enough and now his feet are in the water!"

Lee's and Curt's stories show that they both have significant difficulty comprehending emotional expression as well as narrative. It's not surprising that the two difficulties appear together. The emotional content of every human story is just as important to its making sense as the actions that weave together to form a plot. Lee and Curt don't really get what's going on with the characters depicted in the story-picture I showed them, and they probably can't entirely figure out what's going on in the stories that unfold around them, involving family members, classmates, or strangers. What may be worst of all for them, though, is that they may not understand themselves. Narrative is precisely what is required of each one of us as we piece together the experiences of our lives into a story that makes sense to us. Without the ability to meaningfully integrate observations and experiences, our perception of self, and reality in general, is fragmented, confusing, and stressful.

As nine-year-old Riley stood in the lunch line of his school cafeteria, he tried hard to take in all the comments whirling around him. He mistakenly felt those comments were directed at him, and his inability to stop them or make sense of what he was hearing only fueled his anxiety and frustration. (The intensity of Riley's self-consciousness caused him to miss other essential cues that would have helped him put what he was hearing in context.) Finally, Riley gave in to his stress and pushed another child. Immediately, the line erupted into chaos, and about fifteen minutes later Riley found himself sitting across the desk from his school principal. When the principal asked, "Why did you push another student?" Riley looked dumbfounded. He was so angry that the other students were not being punished for what he had perceived as mockery that his eyes welled up with tears as he pondered the principal's question.

▪ ▪ ▪
The Power of Narrative
Psychologists have observed that even people who sustain severe trauma are better able to cope when they are good historians of the events in their lives. When a boy is able to describe his experiences, his words and memories are the threads that weave disparate events into the cohesive fabric of his life's story. For example, a child who is the victim of bullying needs to talk about what has happened to him, but a boy who can go beyond mere facts, to describe how he felt about being bullied, has the best chance of moving past that conflict in a psychologically healthy way.

Making the Most of Learning and Memory

Many boys have to be taught repeatedly to relate words to experiences, and this process is most effective when it begins early in life. When a child's mental map for a particular event or experience is formed, an emotional state is neurologically linked with that map or memory. Psychologists often refer to this link between a situation and an emotion as *state-dependent learning.* What this means is that various aspects of an experience—such as images, sounds, and sensations—will be encoded in a person's memory and linked with the specific emotional states that occurred during the experience. Remarkably, recalling specific experiences will often bring back the same emotional states. Think about the first time you fell in love. Chances are, the better you can recall the sights and sounds that you perceived at that time, the more clearly you can remember how you felt.

Positive emotional development can be thought of as a sequence of constructive links between life experiences and the thoughts and feelings we have in response to those experiences. *For parents who are committed to nurturing emotional well-being, the goal is to make constructive interpretations and healthy behavior increasingly automatic.* With repeated rehearsal, most behavior becomes more reflexive, sometimes to the extent that it appears intuitive. Just as your hands and fingers move more smoothly after years of piano lessons, a boy's reflexive thoughts and communication will reflect what he has learned and practiced.

Children develop in response to their environments (which includes communication), and your actions and their home and school life constitute that environment. Children are better able to *choose* positive behavior if they are shown how to enact that possibility at a young age. Boys who are neglected, or have their tentative impulses toward positive emotional behaviors repressed or ignored, will have a more difficult time experiencing a healthy respect for self and others as they mature. Let me also suggest that someone who is emotionally literate is better equipped to appreciate and respond independently to life's opportunities. When seventeen-year-old Rodney learned that his basketball team's leading scorer would be out for the season, he immediately felt a twinge of stress and resignation. Looking around at his other teammates, he could see they felt the same. Spontaneously, Rodney said, "Guys, we're feeling sorry for ourselves. I'll be the first to admit I'm shook, but there's no way we can justify giving up. Let's just get it out of our system—who wants to sound off?" Emotional literacy doesn't have to sound like a self-help book or even necessarily be eloquent, but it does imply an awareness of one's feelings and, often, the ability to use those feelings to lead others.

Some parents spend more time teaching their sons how to do algebra than how to greet a friend, behave in a group, or constructively assert an opinion. Statistically, relatively few boys will be required to use algebra as adults, but all boys will have to accomplish social tasks in their daily lives as adults. Of course, there is merit in mastering algebra, but we should adopt a proportional perspective of childhood learning, emphasizing the teaching of those skills that will have the most impact on a person's quality of life in adulthood.

Paying Attention to Nonverbal Cues

Another important dimension of communicating and experiencing emotions is related to *qualities of speech*. By this I mean that the tone, speed, volume, and pitch of voice are neurologically linked with encoded mental images and memories. Most parents learn to effectively redirect children by shifting the tone or volume of their speech. (Lowering one's voice and using a child's middle name is a well-known strategy!) In a similar manner, children interpret the disposition of parents and other authority figures through subtle nuances of speech and expression. These cues may also include physical gestures and facial expressions. All of these factors conspire, helping children to generate an interpretation and conclusion about another person's emotional state. Boys have consistently more difficulty in correctly interpreting these types of clues than do girls, a topic we'll discuss in detail in Chapter 7. The rapid evolution of social change, including an increasingly crowded planet, has made sensitivity to expressive nuances more critical today than at any time in human history. There is no question that boys can learn these skills effectively. Consider the multilayered nuances of music videos, elaborately encoded with signs for the initiated. My point is that emotional literacy has different dimensions and that our sons draw on diverse perceptual skills to learn the language of emotions.

It is important for boys to be encouraged and challenged to express themselves, including the unique and idiosyncratic insights that help them differentiate themselves from others. Boys whose parents seek opportunities to gently nudge more in-depth communication of ideas will develop greater verbal dexterity and improve their verbal memory. In turn, they will be better prepared to learn and understand new words, phrases, and syntax. When we ask boys to express and clarify what they feel, we help them refine and expand their emotional vocabulary.

When challenged, boys may surprise themselves, as their memories can help them pull for words that were stored in their consciousness but seldom retrieved. After hurricane Isabel ravaged the Chesapeake Bay, my wife and I, accompanied by our then two-year-old son, traveled to the bay to inspect the status of our boat. We arrived just after nightfall, and our dock was seriously damaged. Despite a precarious situation, I was determined to climb over the debris and check the boat. As I got out of the truck with my wife's strong warning to "be careful," my son, who had been unusually quiet for several minutes, suddenly burst out, "I'm worried!" I had not heard him say that word in any previous situation, nor had I ever heard him so overtly express anxiety, but it was clear that the phrase and emotional tone were available to him when he needed to convey strong feelings. If he had never been taught the word *worry*, he might have felt blocked in his ability to express what he was feeling. When we build our sons' vocabulary for emotions, we are preparing them to be expressive and active participants in all kinds of life experiences.

When your son loses a game of chess with you, and you can see that he's upset, ask him if he's mad about losing, hates losing to *you*, or just frustrated that he isn't getting better as fast as he thought he would. And if he wins a game, and joyfully proclaims his satisfaction, try expanding his emotional vocabulary with relevant terms; is he exhilarated, triumphant, proud, excited, surprised, honored? One more subtle technique is to scaffold your son's vocabulary by using syn-onyms yourself. One father said to his eight-year-old, "I'm frustrated the Yankees lost; it's exasperating." His son knew the word *frustrated* well enough to draw some pretty solid ideas about what *exasperating* means, especially when put in a helpful learning context.

■　■　■

I hope our exploration of boys of few words has shown you how important communication is to a boy's development. Boys have as much to say as girls, but for both psychological and neurological rea-sons the task can be much harder for them. We have also seen how the resistance to communication some boys display requires sensitiv-ity, skill, and patience on the part of parents. Nowhere is it more im-portant for you to persevere than in helping your son learn the lan-guage of emotions. It can quite literally mean the difference between illness and health over the course of a lifetime. When we teach our sons how to express empathy, we nurture that reflex deep within their minds and give them a tool to enrich the great variety of relation-ships life has to offer.

As promised, Part II will explore psychological and neurodevelop-mental obstacles that often make achieving competent communica-tion and emotional literacy difficult for boys. We'll discuss the chal-lenges and complexities of helping boys who are shy and withdrawn, angry and resistant, and boys whose brain differences make social communication more difficult. Our goal will have less to do with cat-egorizing boys than with better understanding that the road to healthy social development may be obstructed in more than one way. Your own son may be a composite of two or more of the challenging types of boys I will discuss. Boys can be angry and shy, or withdrawn and impulsive. When we are willing to see our sons with open eyes, we are one critical step closer to being the parents they need us to be.

Part II

Especially Challenging Boys

...

FIVE

Encouraging Shy
and Withdrawn Boys

■ ■ ■

Childhood and adolescence are times of rapid transition. As each period of development unfolds, new challenges emerge, accompanied by the demand to master new skills. Growing up is hard enough, but having to "change" in front of others makes it even tougher, especially for boys, whose self-image of competence often rests on *not* changing. Boys need poise and courage to deploy new words to accomplish diverse social missions, to take risks in self-expression, and to stand fast during the barrage of peer reactions that punctuate childhood and adolescence. And these efforts are critical to boys' developing the social communication skills that will serve them throughout life. As parents, we help them through the fears that could otherwise inhibit their social growth.

I believe most of us could agree that the fear of rejection is one of the most potent anxieties a person can experience. Anticipating rejection can quickly undermine a boy's self-confidence, limit healthy risk taking, and, if strong enough, send him scurrying into his shell. With the best of intentions, we encourage our sons to "just say it," or "go ahead, she (he) won't bite." But boys know better. They have learned from a young age that the reactions and remarks of some peers do bite. Every time they could or should communicate, they have to weigh the benefits of making their private selves known against the costs of leaving themselves open to attack and, possibly, emotional injury. In some cases, when boys are especially shy, social communication takes true courage. So, we parent our shy sons best when we en*courage* them, helping them transform an instinct for avoidance into a plan for participation.

Boys can become excessively shy or withdrawn for a variety of reasons. Sometimes shyness stems from temperament and personality. We may notice these traits in our sons at a very early age as they struggle with meeting new people or in making themselves part of a group. But shyness can also develop or intensify as the result of social experiences, including awkward communication. Some boys become so self-conscious about what to say, or how their communication is perceived, that they withdraw socially, feeling as though it's their only option for emotional safety. As parents, we need to know how to make these distinctions about our sons. What we might prematurely chalk up to a boy's personality may in fact be a kind of learning challenge that requires at least as much guidance as it does emotional support.

Boys Who Don't Know *How* to Participate Socially

Griffin, tall and thin at age eleven, lives in a condominium complex with few other families. "There aren't many 'natural' opportunities for him to socialize," his mother explains, "so we have to arrange get-togethers with friends or extracurricular activities. But I'm always the one initiating a plan—I suggest signing up for a club or I call up my sister to get him together with his cousins. Unfortunately, he doesn't seem to develop a social life of his own. He's a nice boy, and people like him well enough, but he's so quiet and shy. He's physically present but is always on the outside of things. He just doesn't know how to join in. If I wasn't orchestrating his friendships, I think people would forget all about him. Maybe he'd be just as content if I stopped trying—I don't know. I've suggested that he pick up the phone and call a classmate, and I keep trying to guess what kind of activity will interest him, but he just shrugs. Then he mopes around home and complains that he has nothing fun to do."

Sound familiar? If you have a son who is exceedingly shy, you might know what social awkwardness like Griffin's looks like. The social experiences of shy, withdrawn boys have sensitized them to the perils of novel situations, and they have opted for withdrawal as a strategy for reducing emotional risk—costly though it may be. Social language does not come easily to these boys, and they have learned that peers can be harsh in responding to their insecurities. Griffin's mother had the right instincts—that he needed more opportunity for exposure and practice in social situations. However, it was apparent that he wasn't ready to jump in and participate socially at the level of his peers. "Is Griffin more communicative with you and your husband?" I asked. "Somewhat," she replied. "He tends to be a quiet boy, but somehow it feels more relaxed and companionable when it's just the three of us. He likes to play cards and board games with us. When others are around, I just feel this anxiety coming from him."

We decided on a multipronged plan to get Griffin's social communication development back on track. First, Griffin would get some coaching from his parents to become more expressive in the nonthreatening environment of his home. When you have a "low-maintenance" child like Griffin, it's easy to settle into a comfortable routine that may not stimulate your son to grow socially. So I loaned Griffin's parents a catalog of board games used by therapists that rely on communication and suggested that, rather than spending meals reading, they pick a topic for discussion. Even though it might feel awkward or "artificial" at first, this kind of contrivance can be an important demonstration to your son of how important you believe communication skills are. And it's especially effective when you already have a good relationship with your son and he's eager to please you.

▪ ▪ ▪
Nonthreatening Peers Can Help

If your son is shy or socially awkward, you can help him by expanding his range of possible playmates to include those who will be compatible and encouraging. Your son may be more comfortable with friends who:

- Are chronologically younger but socially comparable
- OR are old enough to be less competitive or less impatient with him
- Are sunny-tempered and calm (especially for anxious boys)
- Are female or involve him in coed play groups

As a boy develops practice in social situations where his chances for success are maximized, it will help build his courage to expand his set of friends. Have you noticed if there are friends or siblings who bring out the best (or worst) in your son?

We also decided it might be helpful for Griffin to begin socializing more within the relative safety of his home and with a younger child whose social skills more closely matched his own. Griffin's mother strategically invited her eight-year-old nephew, Cal, to their home on a weekly basis. After a while, they resumed visiting all of Griffin's cousins at their house. "At first Griffin followed Cal around like a lost puppy, but you could see that the time he had spent with Cal was like a bridge to help him get involved with his older cousins," his mother said. "My sister has been really helpful too. She thinks that once he's really comfortable joining in with her kids, she'll invite one or two boys in from the neighborhood, so Griffin gets used to playing with someone other than family."

Boys Who Feel Most Capable in the Realm of the Mind

For other boys, avoidance of socializing grows from a personality oriented toward the intellectual realm, a place where ideas and introspection trump the rewards of social interaction. Kevin, a heavy-set twelve-year-old with a mass of curly black hair and a naturally intense facial expression, was a math wizard.

"How do you get along with the other kids at school?" I asked him.

"They think I'm weird. A brain, but weird," he replied frankly.

"Does that bother you?" I asked.

"Not really," he replied. "The truth is, I'm a lot more advanced than they are."

The confident aloofness of boys like Kevin can be very convincing. The fact that they feel competent intellectually can encourage them to put up a self-assured front that this is all they need in life. It's only when you get to know them well that you see the signs of social yearning, and even then you might have to be very alert.

Whether because of social anxiety or social aloofness, the boys described in this chapter are bound by internal walls. Rather than embracing social development, they learn to "cope with it" by minimizing social risk. Again, there's nothing wrong with personality traits of shyness or aloofness. The trouble is, when combined with boys' inherent communication challenges, these traits may discourage boys from socializing to the point where they become socially and emotionally detached. When this is the case, you can be sure they need a helping hand.

For Kevin, the opportunity to build social skills occurred at a summer camp program for some of the nation's brightest young students. For the first time, he found other kids who had similar interests, many of whom were "outsiders" at their home schools. He made some friends, and the following year at school he was less inclined to be condescend-

▪ ▪ ▪

Reading a boy's mind is anywhere from difficult to impossible, but some important questions to consider in determining whether your son is becoming socially adrift include:

- Are your questions met with a stare of detachment, as if he doesn't know why you're asking *him* this?
- Are all or most of his favorite activities solitary?
- Do you notice that peers seem confused about how to relate to him?
- Does he seem to be alone by choice or default?

ing or distant among his classmates. Building on a newfound sense of confidence in his social potential, and with the encouragement of a teacher, Kevin formed a math team in his middle school. He enjoyed the unexpected opportunity to be something of a role model to the other kids and was able to let his defenses down enough to be helpful rather than patronizing. Instead of seeing his difference as a liability, he began to use his special talent as an asset to connect with others.

Above It All—*Including* Others?

When shy boys avoid socializing, they may seem indifferent or even as if they feel superior. For many boys—like Kevin—this takes the form of behaving like intellectuals, individuals who are above the vagaries of emotions and deal only in reason. Usually they are attempting to compensate for feelings of social inadequacy by projecting higher than reasonable self-confidence. Jacob, a shy sixth-grader, responded this way when asked about his friends: "Well, I don't usually make friends. I don't like to have to talk to them, and the way they joke and laugh makes them look kind of stupid." Later, he admitted that he would like to have a special friend or two but didn't know how to go about finding one. Even then, he worked hard to keep the concern on an intellectual plane, giving the impression it wasn't that big a deal. "If they want to be my friends, then fine, but I need time for other things too."

Sometimes boys will compensate for their con-

■ ■ ■

Intellectualizing is a preferred defense for smart, shy boys. By discussing personal matters on a purely "logical" basis, they avoid the uncomfortable emotions associated with their growth and development.

cerns about social exclusion with fantasies of being special in an unusual way. Amal, a third-grader who was small for his age, sat swinging his legs on a chair in my office. Gravely, he told me, "I'm too old for the kids in my class, but they need me to make decisions. I'll probably be their boss when we're all grown up." When I asked Amal about his teacher's observation that he had difficulty getting the attention of peers, he replied, "See, that's what I mean: they could use me to make decisions, but they won't let me tell them. I think someone is going to have to tell the kids in my class to listen to me."

When boys attempt to compensate for social anxiety by asserting some type of superiority or social indifference, we parents have a tough balancing act to perform. It's natural to be concerned about the accuracy of our sons' appraisal of social situations or the possibility that they'll use distorted beliefs as a justification for increasingly greater social withdrawal. Still, we should not necessarily be in a hurry to rid boys of the psychological buffer that helps to preserve the integrity of their self-esteem—even when we perceive that self-esteem is unjustifiably inflated! As discussed, a boy's search for personal mastery runs parallel to his search for self-worth, and when we deflate the former, the latter will also suffer. Deconstructing the walls of deception requires enduring, unconditional love and support. Only in providing this emotional foundation can we hope to help boys consider removing their masks of invulnerability.

Keaton and His Imaginary Band

Keaton, a ninth grader at a competitive high school, played electric guitar and had his own "band." His father thought his grades could be better and that he spent too much time fantasizing about becoming a rock star. "He says he's going to be famous, but he quit guitar lessons after a year. He can play some basic chords, but he really spends more time talking about his band than practicing. That's another issue—he's talked to a couple of other boys about starting a band, but nothing seems to get going. He says they weren't good enough, but as far as I know he can hardly play himself!" I asked how Keaton was doing in school. "He was a good student through seventh grade. But that was a much smaller school, and now he has a lot of competition. His grades have slipped to average, and his teachers say it's mostly because he doesn't participate in class. I try talking to him, but all he can say is everything is boring." His father and I considered a range of possibilities—was the schoolwork too easy or too challenging? Was he having social problems in the classroom? I asked Keaton's father to talk to some of his teachers and try to get a more accurate picture of what was happening in school. He said the teachers felt Keaton was capable of doing the work. What struck Keaton's father most was that "some teachers seemed to have a hard time describing him socially." He wondered if Keaton was really getting noticed. "Maybe that's what he wants," he said.

The key to understanding Keaton came from an unconventional source. His mother was on a committee with another woman whose daughter Tara was at Keaton's school. She asked her friend if her daughter knew Keaton and if she could find out what the other kids thought about her son. "I told Tara to tell me the truth—she wouldn't hurt my feelings. According to Tara, the other kids think Keaton is a mystery. Most of the time he's quiet, but he's also shown he can be argumentative, especially if someone challenges his opinions or the way he wants to do something. I can see that, because I sometimes have the same problem with Keaton. It's like he's hurt if you disagree with some things—not all things, just those things that for whatever reason are very important to him. Tara gave me the feeling that other kids were a little freaked out by him."

"Could his interest in music help?" I inquired.

"It might, but we heard Keaton was telling people he had a band, and some other students challenged him to prove it, which of course he couldn't. I'm sure he feels humiliated, but I'm worried that if I ask him about it he'll feel worse. It seems like the key to his whole identity is tied up in this rock star thing. We don't want to go along with a delusion, but we don't want to discourage or embarrass him more either."

His parents decided on a new tactic. His father said, "We told him we would be proud to support his dream, but we thought he needed a realistic plan to achieve it. We have a small barn out back, and we said we'd help him set up a studio and get him some professional equipment if he did three things: resume his guitar lessons, find some band members he could work with, and get his grades up. If he did that, we agreed that at the end of the year we would consider letting him transfer to another school if he's still feeling bad about things. The thing is, we made it clear that we had to see an honest effort before we would consider an 'evacuation plan.'"

"It was an uphill battle at first. He just wasn't moving forward at a rate we thought was acceptable," his mother commented. "I had this picture in my mind that we'd be back where we started, the barn just a barn and Keaton plucking at his guitar alone in his room. But then we lucked out—we found a guy who gives lessons and has been a studio musician for some big names. We brought Keaton over, and it was like a light went on for him. This guy was telling him about how these session players work in the studios, telling him some stories about the musicians. Keaton felt special just knowing this guy. Even if he never gets to that level, it seems like a fantastic goal for him to aspire to. He's applying himself in a way we've never seen before."

I asked what impact this was having at school. Keaton's father offered, "He's doing all right. His grades have gone up, and we're encouraging him to work *with* the other boys in his band. The biggest thing is that he's a little more receptive to hearing advice. He sees us as believing in him rather than trying to control him, because he's gotten out of that negative rut. Before, he was holding everyone at arm's length because he didn't have any real sense of achievement— it was all a front."

Keaton was able to relinquish his inflated opinion of himself and allow himself to be vulnerable enough to join in relationship with others when he was required to take concrete steps toward achieving a realistic goal. Not every parent has the resources that Keaton's parents do, but every family can replicate the steps they took to help their son out of alienation and withdrawal. First, they thoroughly investigated the probable causes of his problem, including ruling out academic challenges with his teachers and using their network for social support (in their case, friends and a psychologist). Second, they planned an intervention, which they initiated with loving support. The intervention had both positive incentives for achievement and negative consequences for further withdrawal. Third, they were flexi-

▪ ▪ ▪

What do you do when your son is so shy or withdrawn that it affects your family or impairs his potential for happiness or success? A successful plan for helping shy or withdrawn boys involves the following steps:

- Thoroughly investigate probable causes of your son's withdrawal, including the type of learning and attention problems discussed in Chapter 7.
- Consider the impact of school.
- Use the insight and advice of those around you, including other family members, friends, teachers, or professionals.
- Initiate any interventions with loving support.
- Provide appropriate positive incentives and negative consequences.
- Be flexible and creative.

ble and creative. Although their primary goal was to help their son in school, they worked with his primary area of interest—music—to build a bridge to success.

Looking for Signs That a Boy Wants to Connect

Have you ever been around someone so shy that you started feeling anxious yourself? That is what happened to me the first time I met Warren, a nineteen-year-old whose mother had called me to ask if I could help with his social anxiety. Warren was a student at a nearby college, and the first time I met him I could sense his fear and apprehension. He could barely bring himself to make brief eye contact, holding his body tight and stiff. Warren's anxiety about coming to see me was so palpable that his fear instilled within me some of the same awkwardness he was obviously feeling. Reflecting on that meeting, I am somewhat amazed that Warren continued to schedule sessions, but he did, compelled by his growing need to evolve from the anxiety that had disabled his social development for so long. During my work with Warren I learned that social anxiety had shaped many of his most important decisions, including choosing a single room within his dormitory, eating at low-traffic times in the college cafeteria, and rarely leaving his room except to attend class.

■ ■ ■

Many shy boys send signals that they want us to reach out to them, but those signals are rarely verbal. Shy boys who want to connect prefer the listening role, and although they may struggle to take their turns leading a conversation, they will be good listeners for as long as you let them. Other signals worth noting are a desire to be in physical proximity with others, even if they aren't verbally relating. For very shy boys, basic physical inclusion in a group or activity may decrease their often incessant worry about how shyness affects their lives. A good strategy when you see this type of behavior is to bring your observation into the "here and now." Let your son know you've noticed he's shy. Perhaps disclose how you dealt with an experience of shyness at his age, and maintain a relaxed, problem-solving attitude. This will be a message of reassurance that you can work through his problems with him—at a pace that feels safe.

Warren's challenges highlight how shyness leads boys to become unduly self-conscious, particularly with regard to peer acceptance. Lacking confidence and social intuition, they "freeze" when confronted with social situations. Almost always, they find themselves at a loss for words. The basic process of exchanging hellos, making small talk about one's day, and knowing how to "sign off" from social conversation is a tremendously confusing affair for boys like Warren. Because of social anxiety, Warren worked hard to avoid situations that would heighten his fear and self-consciousness. However, he rarely stopped worrying about getting caught in those situations unexpectedly. Withdrawal and avoidance were Warren's primary strategies for averting social stress.

What too often happens with boys like Warren is that we assume they've made a clear choice about how to live their lives. The front of social indifference is so solid that we buy into the ruse that nothing is lacking and leave them alone. Yet if we look closer, taking the time to know such boys, we will often see that what looks "chosen" is actually a boy's best available default. I believe such boys are sending us signals for help all the time, but we miss those signals because they get expressed in convoluted ways. Perhaps we shouldn't be surprised when boys with expressive challenges are challenged to express their problem!

When Social Awkwardness Comes Out Aggressively

Most shy boys are socially awkward, but not all socially awkward boys come across as shy. They may, however, withdraw just like more recognizably shy boys when their attempts to socialize are unsuccessful. Socially awkward elementary school age boys are caught in a conundrum: to risk rejection or miss out on the group fun. Struggling with this dilemma, younger boys may behave or communicate erratically. When these boys talk to other children, their anxiety may cause them to express themselves in a manner that comes across as impulsive or even rude.

Mitchell, a shy eight-year-old, developed a habit of disrupting his class and making social interaction among classmates uneasy. He tended to stay on the periphery of social groups, but his teacher noticed that he watched classmates very closely. Her experience with second graders suggested to her that Mitchell wanted to be a part of the group but lacked the confidence necessary to join in the spontaneous and relaxed interplay. Mitchell began alienating his peers even further, with behavior like what she described in a note to his guidance counselor: "Mitchell upset two boys in class who were playing

■ ■ ■

Does your son tend to blurt out comments in the midst of group discussions, taking everyone by surprise and appearing to interrupt? Does he go on and on about a subject that his listeners don't seem to care about, oblivious to their lack of interest? This can be the manifestation of shyness, as much as it seems like the opposite. I have seen many socially awkward boys lose their composure and say the first thing that comes to mind. I've seen others get so charged with anxiety that they're on a "runaway train" and can't get off. Unfortunately, many of these boys privately tend to obsess about their social ineptitude, particularly as they reach the middle school years. After an embarrassing interlude, they "play back" the conversation to themselves and are even less likely to speak up at the next social gathering. Part of the art of parenting such boys is to balance the need to redirect their behavior with an understanding that the words we choose will linger in their minds. "Terrence, it's great to see you so excited, but let's listen to what Erica wants to say" is better than "Terrence, enough, give someone else a chance."

checkers. He began to point out the moves and became angry when they complained. He then called them names and began to cry. Please help Mitchell understand when and how to join in with other students."

Social anxiety can bring about a high level of internal pressure, causing a boy to feel as if he must quickly find a way to discharge that stress. Understandably, this kind of stress impairs judgment about the timing and tone of self-expression. And the choices boys make can be misread as being competitive, aggressive, or just plain thoughtless.

Unfortunately, we can't just talk boys out of listening to the anxiety that makes them turn inward. We can, however, give them the tools they need to feel competent instead of fearful and gently encourage them to use them. Our best chance of positively impacting shy boys is to show them how to navigate social communication hurdles through example and opportunity. One important way to do so is to provide concrete examples about how to communicate socially and let them observe our words and deeds.

■ ■ ■

Parents as Trainers

At times, you may actually need to shadow your son as he works to make an introduction, form a conversation, or simply cope with the presence of a large group of peers. You may need to coach your child on the specifics of saying hello and meeting people, using appropriate facial expressions and gestures to convey meaning, or provide sample "scripts" he can use in different social situations.

When It Doesn't Come Naturally, Teach

J.J., an introverted four-year-old, had moved with his parents, Ben and Christine, to a new neighborhood. "One of the reasons we bought the house was that there are so many kids nearby. Our yards all back to a community green, and there's a playground in the middle. When Ben takes him to the playground, J.J. wants his dad to climb on the equipment with him. He won't go off and play with the other kids," Christine explained.

"He won't even let go of my hand!" laughed Ben, "and I'm too big for the slides."

"How have you helped him?" I asked.

"Well, we encourage him to go play with the other kids, tell him that they're nice, let him know that we'll be right there on the benches watching him," said Christine.

"Suppose this happened to you," I said. "You joined a new company, an international conglomerate involved in important business with the governments of several nations. As part of your duties, you'd be flying to a foreign country and meeting with the prime minister and his deputies at a state event. As you enter the reception hall, your colleague tells you that he'll be joining the minister of finance at her table but suggests that you cultivate some of the other dignitaries—wonderful people—who are present. You've never been to this country and are unfamiliar with its customs. How would you feel?"

Ben and Christine laughed. It's easy to forget that what looks like a fun new playground to an adult could look like intimidating foreign territory to a young child.

For some children, the unfamiliar evokes more fear and anxiety than curiosity and excitement. J.J. was going to need a course in "diplomatic relations" to develop the confidence necessary to join the other children. If you were going to that diplomatic reception, you would want a briefing on the event, some tips on what to say and how to say it, and probably would appreciate an advance introduction to some of the people there so you wouldn't feel like a complete stranger. In the same way, J.J.'s parents could help him by preparing him for the playground. "Get a book about making friends, practice making introductions, and let him see you meeting people as well," I suggested. "Perhaps you could go up to another parent and child and say something like 'Hi, I'm Ben and this is J.J.' You're likely to get a friendly response and a return introduction, so you could mention that you're new in the neighborhood and that J.J. likes the slides, maybe get into a conversation with the other parent or child about what he likes to do. You could then ask J.J. questions to stimulate social thinking and banter, or walk over to some play equipment together so that he can be near the other child but have the reassurance of your presence. If he does well with this, on the walk home praise him for doing such a good job. If he finds it difficult, you can offer some gentle suggestions about what he can try next time—it could be as simple as saying, 'You could try smiling at the other kids so they'll know how friendly you are.'"

After a few weeks I asked Ben and Christine how it was going.

"It's going pretty well. There were a few awkward moments. J.J. had practiced saying 'Hi, I'm J.J., do you want to play with me?' at home, and when we went to the playground he went up to a younger boy and said 'Hi, I'm J.J. Do-you-wanna-play-with-me?' and the other boy didn't know what to do and ran away. So we had to explain that he was too little to understand him and coach J.J. to try again," his parents said.

In the meantime Christine had met another mom, who invited them over to play with her daughter. "It was kind of funny. J.J. walked right in and used the same line—'Hi, I'm J.J. Do-you-wanna-play-with-me?'—and the other mother exclaimed, 'Oh, isn't he so cute!' and the girl just took his hand and led him to the toys, so that went well. Then we set up a time for him to go with her to the playground. I think having a 'script' is reassuring to him, so every time before we go somewhere, we tell him some things that he can say. It's helped a lot," Ben said.

Practicing the Communication Code

Becoming good at communicating requires that a boy have lots of practice speaking, gaining comfort with the sound of his own voice and learning how the subtleties of his voice convey meaning. Most of us can identify with situations in which we might feel nervous about speaking in front of a group or to people who might judge us. But for some boys of few words, social fear dominates their relationships with peers and adults and can occur in situations many of us would consider benign or encouraging.

Often a boy like this is quiet, reluctant to let the sound of his voice be heard. Elliot, a very bright eleven-year-old, cannot bring himself to raise his hand in class because he blushes and his voice warbles when called on by his teacher. He is already learning to weigh the advantages of emotional safety against the value of demonstrating his intelligence. Logan, an athletically built and seemingly popular thirteen-year-old, is so self-conscious he complains frequently, "Other kids are always staring at me." His anxiety causes him to constantly feel as if he has to check for what he's doing wrong. His parents worry that he "acts like a stone" to avoid any possible interpretation of his thoughts or feelings by others.

Like the angry and resistant boys we'll talk about in the next chapter, shy and avoidant kids often suffer from inadequate practice in communicating. Their social anxiety makes it so painful for them to interact that they'll go to great lengths to avoid situations in which they will be required to express themselves.

Despite the extraordinary challenges some children have had to face in their lives, they have a reasonably good chance to overcome social hurdles if they're able to interpret their social deficits as skills they have simply yet to learn. To help boys consider this perspective, it's helpful to present the task of overcoming their challenges as learning a code. The notion of a code refers to a kind of secret knowledge that, once learned, can potentially open doors.

Byron is nine. Before his parents divorced when he was two, his mother apparently yelled at him often, and his father feels that those early experiences caused him to be shy and withdrawn. His ultimate goal was to make a friend and invite him over to his house to play.

> ∎ ∎ ∎
>
> **Crack the code . . .**
> Behaviors as basic as extending a hand for a handshake, giving compliments, or asking follow-up questions to someone's statement are part of the social communication code. Although we hope that boys will ultimately use these skills more reflexively, they will need prompting to get those social reflexes jump-started.

During our first meeting, I asked Byron if he knew the code for how to do that. His curiosity about this mysterious code was the foundation for our therapeutic partnership, a lure that parents can use as well.

As with Griffin, who had to learn to communicate socially one step at a time—first at home with just his parents, then with his younger cousin, then with his older cousins too, and finally with the cousins' friends—the best way to teach the communication code is a little at a time. We started with the basics—Byron practiced making eye contact and saying hello in my office. But he didn't start practicing with me; he started by talking to a Lego man we built together. In my office there are shelves of toys and games, and for many boys construction toys provide a strategic distraction that facilitates more relaxed discussion of the challenges that bring them to therapy. Eventually, we built a space station and I advised Byron that the captain of the space station liked to be greeted each day. Byron accepted this suggestion and began greeting the yellow-faced Lego man with a hearty "hello" each session. We extended our play to include personal greetings in my waiting room, where I would coach Byron to use both verbal and nonverbal communication. This involved a degree of social risk, since there would often be other people present. His father remarked that at school, although Byron was still not particularly talkative with peers, he had learned how to establish a social connection with his booming "hello."

The next step was for Byron's father and stepmother to coach his social communication during practice with peers. They helped Byron choose and invite peers to come to his house to play, and during those visits he joined the kids in various kinds of games. This gave Byron's parents an opportunity to provide needed reassurance and a chance to model communication skills when they saw Byron needed some guidance. After some time, Byron found one or two consistent friends about whom he loved to chat. He had changed his beliefs about social possibilities through the strategic, loving support of his parents and by practicing elements of the social communication code.

Letting Them Hear You

One thing that parents and teachers of young children should be particularly aware of is how we speak about them in their presence. It always surprises me how many people forget that the object of their assessment is standing before them, ears wide open. "Don't mind him, Charlie's shy" is as much an appraisal as a self-fulfilling prophecy. Even well-meaning advice substantiates the presence of a problem; for highly sensitive boys, the gentlest suggestion can sound like a criticism.

> ■ ■ ■
> Make sure what you say about your son reinforces the positive, letting him "overhear" you praise his good behavior. In addition, refrain from characterizing your son in ways that might provide a "negative script" for his conscious or unconscious understanding of himself.

Challenges for Shy Boys in School

As boys immerse themselves in a community of peers, they come face-to-face with social differences. Even during the first years of elementary school, they can be acutely aware of their social awkwardness, especially when relentless comparison with peers leads to taunting of those with a perceived weakness like shyness. Unfortunately, being targeted in this way can make a shy boy even more self-conscious of poor expressive skills. Seeking refuge from hurtful words and experiences, it's not illogical that boys would tend to withdraw further. The anger they feel at having to be in an environment where they are constantly being forced to face their deficits may surface as a behavioral problem or may go underground, hidden by stoic faces and the guise of indifference.

Because social skills tend to have a reciprocal relationship with academic skills, many withdrawn or shy boys develop a poor attitude toward school that takes a toll on academic performance. Being a social outsider can have such a marked effect on a boy's self-esteem that he may have difficulty relaxing and focusing well enough to learn. Terrell, a chronically anxious fifth grader, spoke very softly when called on at school. His teacher, whose instructional style was naturally loud and gregarious, tried to make a joke and would use a small megaphone to call out, "Terrell, I can't hear you!" The teacher used this technique with other kids too, and usually it made Terrell's classmates laugh. It might have loosened up Terrell as well, were he more resilient. However, Terrell was anxious, sensitive, and perfectionistic. The embarrassment of being cajoled publicly prompted him to start sitting at the back of the room. On a visit to his school, I noticed him sitting with hunched shoulders, trying to make himself look small. His concentration and learning ability were clearly impaired because he was so anxious about the possibility that he might be called on. Rather than focusing on instruction, Terrell was using his intellect to develop elaborate strategies for avoiding attention. Absorbing and retaining information is hard enough, but it's even harder when a boy's disposition is defensive.

Terrell is one of the boys who "disappear" in school. As they withdraw, they can mistakenly be convinced that invisibility is their ally. It doesn't take most shy boys long to figure out that being quiet is a good strategy for avoiding unwanted attention. And a boy who spends his school day being unobtrusive can find it difficult to switch gears and then be conversant at home. You should be concerned if you notice a significant decrease in your son's verbal output, especially when he resists discussing his day in school. His tendency to-

■ ■ ■

Do you get nothing but a shoulder shrug or a monosyllabic answer when you ask your son, "How was your day?" after school? If this represents a change in behavior, talk to your son's teacher and find out if he's suddenly having problems talking at school. But if your son is very young, keep in mind that putting together a cohesive narrative about his day can be cognitively challenging and may require some training. All parents should prepare their sons to answer such questions as early as preschool. Begin by asking specific questions and praising positive responses: "Whom did you sit next to in circle time? [This is a reminder that he sat next to someone and may prompt his attention toward others in the class.] Was it a boy or a girl? [By age three, most children will be able to make gender discriminations.] What did you sing?" Notice that these questions don't have yes-or-no answers. When your son responds, thank him and say something like, "I'm interested in hearing what you did. You're very good at explaining what happens in your school!" Soon your son might be prompting you with, "Would you like me to tell you about my day?"—just as mine did.

ward silence on that subject may well be a sign of a social or emotional adjustment problem that needs your attention.

The Comparisons Only Get Tougher by High School

By high school, many socially anxious boys become even more self-conscious because of an emerging awareness of how they differ from friends and classmates. They have the same need to preserve self-esteem found among their more socially relaxed peers and consequently will avoid situations that undermine their self-confidence. These boys often feel isolated in school. Just walking down the typical noisy school hallway can be difficult for some boys; they fear being noticed, yet feel excluded as well. Although these boys recognize the presence of a social communication code, they do not grasp the mechanics of how that code works. The type of language and communication skills that seem so effortless for other boys eludes them; confusion reinforces their hesitation to communicate.

Dean, a forty-year-old writer, described his high school experience like this: "I was so hyperconscious of myself. You know that story about the fly about to be eaten by a spider? The fly said, 'Before you eat me, can you explain how you walk with all those legs?' As the spider tried to think about how he walked and describe it to the fly, he started to get flustered. He tried to count which foot moved first, and second, and so on, and got himself so confused and tangled up that he fell into a big heap, and the little fly got away. Well, I was like that spider. If I thought someone was looking at me, I could barely get down the hall without walking into something. And so everyone thought I was a 'spaz'—that was the slang, for 'spasmatic,' I think. Definitely not cool. And I was smart, but I could not open my mouth to talk in class. There was a girl I was totally, unbelievably in love with. She was in most of my classes, and I'm sure she hardly noticed me. But everything—everything—I did in class was a performance, in my mind, for her. How I sat at my desk, the expression on my face, how many notes I took—you name it, I was thinking about how she would perceive it. I could not raise my hand in that class, because I couldn't deal with the lack of control involved in speaking out loud. Plus, I was one of the 'losers.' As soon as one of us got called on, there'd be this little ripple around the class. I don't know if it's anything the teacher would have picked up on, but it definitely broadcast to the other kids, like 'Nerd alert! Nerd alert!' People would shift around in their seats, there'd be these little smirks or, worse, sympathetic smiles on their faces, and after you'd answer, depending on how strict the class was, there'd either be little eye rolls, or mumbled derogatory comments. It was awful."

"How did you deal with it?" I asked.

"Oh, all the wrong ways," Dean admitted cheerfully. "I started drinking, pretty heavily by eleventh grade. When I got drunk, I was uninhibited and said things that other kids thought were funny. It was strange—by my senior year I had developed a reputation as being some kind of cool rebel. It was total bullshit because I was still terrified of being judged. When I went to college, I guess I compensated for my insecurities by continuing to be this 'party guy.' By my sophomore year in college I was on academic probation. It really wasn't until grad

■ ■ ■

If your son's shyness or withdrawal is intensified by a particular situation or environment, it's very important to find a safe place where he can experience social connection. Does your son have a supportive friend, family member, congregation, or social organization he can turn to? How can you encourage him?

school that I figured out I didn't need to put on a mask to find acceptance among my peers. I don't know if anyone could have made me see that sooner, but I sure wish they had tried."

School as a Shocking Transition

Even very young boys can be vulnerable to the impact of school on self-perception. One of the key developmental hurdles young children face is differentiating between family and public domains and learning how to negotiate socially with all kinds of people. Ironically, this transition can initially seem more difficult for boys who are adored by their families or highly protected. Although the love and confidence afforded these boys will likely hold them in good stead, the change in environment can seem shocking.

Younger boys are often noticeably quiet as they navigate the labyrinth of social integration. Parents may be surprised to hear preschool or kindergarten teachers comment on how "quiet" their boys are when they know quite well how conversational their sons can be. It can be difficult for parents to watch their children struggle with the challenges of new social environments like school. It is important to support and thoughtfully reinforce boys through these first attempts at socialization, while their self-concept is still fluid. A child who comes to believe that he is a "social misfit" doesn't come to that conclusion out of the blue; that unfortunate belief stems from early experiences.

Lasting Wounds of Shame

For many boys, the price of being withdrawn is a loss of faith in their social ability. Rather than being perceived as a lack of a skill, social difficulties are accepted as an attribute they'll suffer from forever. William, a shy thirteen-year-old, still remembers with abject humiliation being scolded for hugging a girl in second grade. Rather than saying, "William, we don't grab each other in school, but it's okay to say something nice to Alyssa," an inexperienced teacher's aide had reflexively yanked him away, admonishing him to "quit harassing her." In an apparent effort to make the incident instructive to other students, the aide asked the class if William should be allowed to touch another student. The whole class responded with a resounding "No!" William's mother remembers that for several months after the incident he would complain of having a stomachache. William had physically internalized the idea that he was "bad" for having hugged a girl, and the anxiety was overwhelming for him. Five years later, the image of that humiliation still restricts William's willingness to be expressive.

Socially anxious boys are often plagued by apprehension that keeps them from taking the chances necessary to gain even the most rudimentary social confidence. When they are disciplined, whether at school or at home, it should be clear that the behavior is what needs to be changed, not the boy.

Given how entrenched a boy's self-concept can become, if your son is in an environment that is potentially damaging to his social development, act assertively and quickly. Don't hesitate to work with his teacher, enroll him in a quality social skills course, get him involved in a club where he can apply his talents, or even change schools if your efforts aren't working.

Almost anyone can feel inhibited in new circumstances, and some degree of separation anxiety is normal for young boys. A child who is anxious and worried the first few weeks in school, or who takes some time to make friends, is different from a child who "disappears" in the classroom or is muted by fear. Lyle, a sunny-tempered six-year-old, began protesting going to school when he entered first grade. "At first I thought the transition to a full day was difficult," said his mother. "I called up his teacher, and she said he was very cooperative, a little shy, but she thought he'd do okay. But he was waking in the night with bad dreams and then started wetting the bed. This was all completely new and only occurred when he started school. My mind started racing with all these scenarios, so I called the school again.

"This time the teacher suggested that I come in for a day to help in the class. She said a teacher's aide would sometimes sit at a desk in the back of the classroom, and so it wouldn't seem altogether out of place if I explained to Lyle that I was just helping Mrs. P. with some projects. So I sat in the back cutting out papers and watched Lyle. At first he was very conscious of me and kept turning around to look at me, but I just kept my head down and kept cutting so he'd forget I was there. As I watched Lyle more closely, I saw how intently he would survey the class, hands clasped in front of him, as his teacher had instructed the class to do fifteen minutes earlier. All the other kids had given that up in two minutes. As I watched, I realized that Lyle was very concerned about doing the right thing, following orders. I also noticed that after Mrs. P. said to do something, Lyle quickly looked to the other kids to see what they did and then copied them.

"What I think was happening is that Lyle wasn't used to the fast pace and occasional frenzy of the classroom. He went to a small, private kindergarten where he got tons of individual attention. These kids were all old pros at what happens in school and were adjusted to hearing orders and instructions in rapid succession. They were used to the noise. But I think Lyle was overwhelmed and terrified of making a mistake," his mother said.

"What did you do?" I asked.

"First, I sat down with him and told him a story about how when I was a little girl I had to go to a school where there were too many rules and it was too noisy. I had his full attention! As I told him this story, I asked him if he had any ideas about what helped me," she said. "Lyle said he didn't know, but was very interested in knowing the answer. I told him that my mother had taken me to talk to the teacher to get some ideas together, and that's just what I did with Lyle.

"Mrs. P. was wonderful. I had called her ahead of time, and we had discussed the situation. She told Lyle that she noticed how hard he was working to follow all the rules and thanked him for trying so hard. She told him it would be okay if he made a mistake, but if he had a question he could always raise his hand and ask her. She also told him that if he was feeling very worried he could tug on his ear, and she would give him a secret, friendly message back. So when he did it, she tugged on her ear back and gave him a supportive touch on the head. When his anxiety level went down, he had a much easier time following the class. The bad dreams and bed wetting became much more infrequent."

Caught Up in Their Own Reality

Boys can become so involved in their own thoughts that their shyness develops unconsciously, much like a habit. Especially for cerebral, highly imaginative boys, their internal, mental life can be so captivating that they withdraw from peers. These boys construct private realities that are built around idiosyncratic interests and, frequently, a strong desire to know how things work. Focusing on the structures and components of systems allows socially anxious boys to replace insecurity with a sense of control and safety. As far as it contributes to their self-worth, this is fine. The trouble arises when it crosses the threshold from passion to obsession.

Distinguishing between passion and obsession is not always easy, however, even for parents who know their boys well. Boys who are passionate about their pursuits may infect us with excitement and enthusiasm but are not necessarily inclined to pursue their passion to the exclusion of life's social dimensions. Conversely, obsessions are psychologically limiting. Boys who become obsessed with particular activities or interests may become so caught up that they are unable to set reasonable limits around their degree of involvement in those pursuits. In such cases, boys have arguably become trapped by their own interests and need the help of a parent who can help them more thoughtfully allocate time to a balanced selection of activities.

For shy boys, the possibility of social interest being diverted to an obsession with a system such as mastering games, computers, or even completing a collection is substantial. The challenge of detecting an

■ ■ ■
Passion or Obsession?

Sometimes the intensity of a boy's interest in a hobby or pursuit can cause him to withdraw from other people or activities in his life. For example, most boys enjoy computer games but some can get lost in a "cyber-fantasy world." The difference between a passion and an obsession is that obsessions are psychologically limiting. Some questions to consider about your son's interest or hobby include:

- Does it interfere with his ability to connect with others?
- Does it cause him to lose sleep?
- Does it cause him to lose track of time?
- Is it interfering with his schoolwork?
- Does he spend too much money on it?
- Does he pursue it more during times of stress or to avoid social situations?

If you've answered "yes" to these questions, you may need to help your son achieve a better degree of balance in his life.

obsession is made more difficult by the fact that we expect and hope that boys will be curious about how things work. The intellectual curiosity and concentration of preadolescent boys, especially, can be remarkable. Observed within the context of their individual interests, these boys appear assured. The gaps in self-confidence may not be revealed until they encounter contexts that require interpersonal awareness and social flexibility.

Daniel, a studious and serious twelve-year-old, was about to celebrate his bar mitzvah. His father was concerned about Daniel's ability to recite passages from the Torah before the congregation. When he asked Daniel to practice with him, Daniel didn't respond other than to avoid eye contact. "This is a boy who has memorized every geologic era in the history of the earth. He's quite an amateur scientist. This should be easy for him, but he's determined to fight it," complained his father.

"I don't think Daniel is being defiant. He's always been very interested in Judaism. This problem is that he's terrified to speak in front of so many people," said his mother. "We feel bad for Daniel. He knows his older brothers stood up and spoke beautifully during their bar mitzvahs. Daniel just freezes with a blank look whenever we bring it up, and the clock is ticking."

When the topic of his bar mitzvah was being discussed, Daniel's anxiety was palpable. He looked away, exhaled deeply, and let his shoulders sag. Daniel confided to his brother that he hoped he got seriously ill or had an injury so the bar mitzvah could be called off.

In an effort to ease his anxiety, Daniel's parents began to verbally acknowledge his understanding of the passages he was to read. They worked to make Daniel feel more like a teacher lecturing to others than a student giving a presentation that would be graded. This approach was meant to reinforce his sense of mastery and accomplishment and also gave him an imaginative frame of reference that supported his confidence. "We wanted him to feel like an authority, to help his nerves," his father explained.

His father also casually asked Daniel questions about Judaism before family friends, so that he could become more accustomed to explaining things aloud in the presence of an audience, albeit a small one. Finally, Daniel's father arranged an opportunity with the rabbi to have Daniel practice in the synagogue. Despite Daniel's initial resistance, he was compelled by the encouragement of the rabbi and stood at the podium, speaking in front of his family. "At first he was

■ ■ ■

Practice!

Remind your son that you don't have to be spontaneous to be socially successful. By applying himself, he can improve his communication skills. Some things that can help shy or awkward boys in social situations include:

- Write out a "script" before making a phone call, or keep a "cheat sheet" of responses he can use when he answers the telephone.
- Teach your son acceptable options for verbal "self-defense".
- Prepare and practice before social situations. Especially for younger boys, parents can help their sons anticipate what will happen and coach them on what to say. Role playing helps!
- E-mail can help boys who get tongue-tied in person, because it gives them time to form their words and build confidence in their ability to connect with others. Other forms of writing can help your son's expressive capabilities as well.

so miserable I almost gave up. But our rabbi was very encouraging and gentle and kept cheering him on. What's more, he cleared time from his busy schedule to meet with Daniel several times so that he could get used to standing at that podium," said his father. "This is a man who really doesn't have a spare half hour in his day, and I think Daniel felt supported by such a generous gift of time.

"Just before the bar mitzvah, the rabbi whispered a few words in his ear and gave him a handshake and a pat on the back. Daniel was able to get through it, a little quietly at first, but then much better.

"I asked Daniel what the rabbi said," continued his father. "He simply said that he had complete faith that Daniel could do it and reminded him that his faith was a powerful thing. He understood that Daniel needed a *thought* to hold on to, something to override his emotions. He was able to help Daniel use his faith as a way to overcome his fear, and it is a lesson Daniel is likely to carry with him."

Taking Flight into Fantasy

One particular form of special interest that captivates many boys is science fiction and fantasy. Film series like *Lord of the Rings* and *Star Wars* embody the many myths and rites of passage that shape human experience. Shy boys may be attracted to such stories because it feels easier to experience these passages through art than in life. Unfortunately, if it's only in fiction that boys make such passages, they may not develop the social skills that come along with them.

Fourteen-year-old Kieran, self-proclaimed fantasy fanatic, got involved with a club that played "Dungeons and Dragons," a game based on the stories and myths of the Middle Ages. Kieran's parents were glad that he had found a few friends but noticed that he was increasingly withdrawn and moody, especially after play sessions. They tried to get him to talk about the game and which characters he was playing, but Kieran wasn't very responsive. They discovered that he had been surfing the Internet for sites related to the game, and initially attributed that to his strong interest in fantasy. Shortly thereafter, however, Kieran's parents noticed that he started speaking differently. "It was just little phrases, like 'He's a menace' or 'There are forces beyond our imagination'—it just didn't sound like something he'd normally say," explained his mother. She got concerned when she looked into a school notebook and saw class notes for the beginning of the year, but then nothing but fantasy drawings—things like castles, dragons, and runes. "I don't think he was paying attention to his class, because he got a C in biology, and that's not like him, so I went to the school," said his mother.

"His teachers had also noticed that he was acting different, more distant. We talked about our concern that he was slipping too far into this dungeons fantasy world. Enough is enough. We set up a meeting with Kieran, his teacher, his father and me, and it was fairly constructive. We were assertive in asking him to take a more active role in his classes, or he would have to quit the Dungeons and Dragons club. His teacher also had a great suggestion. He felt that Kieran might benefit from getting involved in some drama because he was so imaginative."

Later, his parents re-

> ■ ■ ■
> ### Three Cheers for the Expressive Arts
> If your son is not a natural speaker, he still needs to find a mode of self-definition. Writing, painting, sculpting, and music all represent alternative modes of communication that can provide him with opportunities for self-reflection and expression. Help your son find a way to get involved. Boys of few words spend altogether too much time as spectators in life.

ported that he had found a new group of friends at school and had become very involved in the school's theater group. "He's had some small roles and really enjoys doing the behind-the-scenes work," they said. "Fortunately, it's collaborative—painting scenes, lighting, and so forth—and we think it's really brought him out. He's found his niche with the 'artsy' kids, where his differences are accepted and his imagination can fly."

The key thing to remember about shy, avoidant, and withdrawn boys is that their social isolation is typically not willful. Consciously or unconsciously, they long for relationships and acceptance. Our job as parents and concerned adults is to help these boys crack the code of social skills and find the self-confidence that will enable them to live lives of greater emotional and social fulfillment. By teaching practical skills and providing a supportive relationship for learning we are helping these boys build the bridges to social competence they need. Our consistent effort in this regard teaches our sons about the importance of perseverance and reinforces the idea that social communication can be learned with patience and practice.

SIX

Reducing the Resistance
of Angry and Antisocial Boys

■ ■ ■

Wong, an eleven-year-old boy who lives with his parents and three sisters, seems to enjoy getting angry and appears to look for things to get irritated about. "I don't know if he wants more attention or if he thinks this is a manly way to talk," said his mother. "He makes a lot of complaints and accuses the girls of things—'You moved my stuff' or 'What are you looking at?' If his sisters argue back, he starts to insult them," she continued. "When we tell him this is not the way to talk, he won't answer us."

Nine-year-old Kelsey has shown that he's capable of behaving very nicely, but he gets terse, rude, or uncommunicative when things aren't going his way. "The other day I came home and his homework wasn't done," said his father, "and he was playing on the computer. I suggested he get his homework done first so he wouldn't have it hanging over his head. Any little suggestion can set him off. He put on his typical sarcastic tone and said, 'No, no, I don't think so.' My partner has more luck because he can joke with him, but I think that's just buying into his bad humor. We shouldn't have to amuse Kelsey so he won't get mad, should we?"

Brandon is a seriously obese fourteen-year-old. At school he shows others that they don't matter to him through a stoic disposition and a cynical communication style. Although his razor-sharp insults protect him from attack, they also insulate him from the possibility of making true friendships. "I don't know how to connect with him anymore," his father complains. "He has a wonderful wit, a great sense of irony, but the fun's gone out of it. His words have a troublesome edge now. It worries me to think about how good Brandon has become at disguising himself. If I didn't know better, I'd be put off by his antics myself."

Six-year-old Enrique has discovered that when he raises his voice at the bus stop, other children become quiet and usually let him put his lunchbox "in line" wherever he wishes. As soon as Enrique gets his way, his voice returns to normal and he interacts with the other children more appropriately. However, his mother is becoming concerned with this type of manipulative outburst, which she sees as Enrique's way of getting what he wants.

The Sounds of Anger . . . and the Many Guises of Antisocial Communication

In the previous chapter you had a chance to explore what might be going on if your son seems shy and withdrawn in his communication and social interactions. Here we're going to consider behavior that often seems like the opposite—the angry, aggressive, sullen, belligerent, or antisocial communication style that is unfortunately fairly common among boys of various ages. This type of behavior is usually very disturbing to parents and can be extremely detrimental to the development of a child's social skills and the relationships that require them.

If Wong, Brandon, Kelsey, or Enrique reminded you of your own son in some ways, you've probably spent a fair amount of time agonizing over the question "What is he so mad about?" I can't promise to lead you to exactly the right answer—there are so many different factors that can account for persistent anger—but it's entirely possible that your son's anger flows from his discomfort with social communication and emotional expression. If that's the core of his problem, this chapter (along with Chapters 8 and 9) will guide you in helping your son make positive changes. But if these interventions don't have a significant, lasting effect, please consult a professional to explore other possible causes of your son's anger (see Chapter 11).

Complicating the challenge of ferreting out the cause of a boy's anger is the fact that the communication of angry boys can take several forms. It may be sharp and assertive, breaking out above the voices of others, or it might be sullen and withdrawn. When angry communication is loud and harsh, you'll probably be able to read its tone quickly and with confidence. Conversely, when angry communication is driven by social retreat, a turning inward, you may feel more ambivalent about what your son is trying to tell you.

What I refer to as "antisocial" behavior in this chapter can also be somewhat confusing to deal with. Although boys exhibiting such behavior don't always appear outwardly angry, their communication tactics reflect poor social adjustment and a drive for control, even domination. This pattern of behavior threatens their healthy social maturation just as do social anxiety, aggressive anger, or the type of neuropsychological problems we will review in the next chapter. Boys who demonstrate antisocial behavior may leave parents and others with an uncomfortable feeling of having been manipulated, put off, or deceived after any individual interaction. Learning to recognize the signs of budding antisocial behavior can help parents to strategically intervene to support their sons' capacity for empathy and emotional literacy. Please understand, however, that the boys described in this chapter are not antisocial in the sense of having a criminal orientation or being sociopathic. Those boys at the far end of the continuum are an extraordinarily complex group that deserve a more in-depth exploration than is possible in this book. When boys of few words are *antisocial*, they are socially resistant for one or more reasons, including being very self-absorbed, sometimes bordering on self-centered. These boys can be so intensely involved in competition and in a need to "win" that they lose sight of the normal give and take of social interaction.

If your son's communication is characterized by anger, your principal goal will be to help him sustain social contact. It's through this contact that you have the best chance of bringing a boy through the stress that often attends anger and helping him find ways to communicate himself out of that anger. Boys do need our help to break an angry pattern of communication. Just as a toddler can sometimes feel an alarming loss of control in the midst of a tantrum and can benefit, alternately, from parental reassurance, redirection, or retreat, there are strategies you can employ with boys of all ages to help them find their way to healthier self-expression. Yet angry boys can be very effective at pushing us away and sometimes cause us to second-guess our understanding of them ("Is something bothering him?"; "Is this a stage?"; "Do all kids talk like this nowadays?"; "Am I taking things too personally?") Sometimes they make us wonder if they actually want to connect. We'll talk about how to break through the walls of anger, helping your son become more comfortable with the vulnerability required to relate and to accept the care of others.

In the case of boys who may tend toward antisocial communication, you'll have a demanding preliminary task: You'll need to tune in a sensitive ear just to identify this problem. Boys of this type often reveal their psychology only through very subtle cues in their speech and language. They may feel especially uncomfortable confiding in adults and acknowledging a sense of personal vulnerability in their relationships with peers. Antisocial boys may be so defensive or verbally manipulative that their communication stays under the radar. It's helpful to remember that the speech of these boys is often defined by resistance to inquiries of a personal nature: "Is everything okay with you?" is answered with "What are you asking me that for? Everything's fine, just back off!" The reply to "What's wrong?" is "Nothing, never mind," or a shrug. In addition, their words are often variations on the themes of domination and competition: "You can't make me" or "I'll tell *you*." What makes your job as a parent more complicated is that these responses can also flow from the natural reticence of some boys or the withdrawal that stems from shyness or anxiety. I hope the many illustrations of different boys offered in this chapter and the previous one will help clarify the difference. Antisocial boys really would rather not connect with you, because their energies are focused elsewhere, they are invested in other psychological goals, or, in some cases, they have underdeveloped interest in, or empathy for, others.

Behind the Anger

Anger can emerge from a variety of causes. As it rises to the surface of a boy's behavior, it's sometimes hard to stop and consider what's motivating his anger. When someone is communicating angrily with you, it usually elicits a strong reaction—whether it's reciprocal anger, anxiety, guilt, or sorrow. When that someone is your son, naturally those feeling are intensified. But if you can step back and determine what's causing his negative communication, you'll be more effectively aligned with those aspects of your son that need your understanding, compassion, and help. Let's look at some reasons your son may have adopted an angry communication style.

Can Your Son Reflect on His Own Emotions and Read Others' Emotions?

Angry communication often sounds and feels aggressive and may be used as a weapon by some boys to fend off feelings of self-consciousness. Research has repeatedly linked aggression with an inability to manage emotions. In a study in the *Journal of Abnormal*

Child Psychology, Dr. Amy Bohnert of Pennsylvania State University found that children with low "emotional competence" were characterized by aggressive behavior. The study's research team noted that aggression was associated with both more intense expressions of unpleasant emotions such as anger and ineffective skills in reading the emotions of others. Bohnert and colleagues also suggest that aggressive children have more difficulty reflecting on their emotional states, particularly in emotionally arousing situations. This study's findings speak to the importance of self-awareness in moderating the effects of anger and aggression, and this is precisely what effective parents can teach their children to do by helping them to verbalize what they are feeling. Sometimes the challenge of developing this skill in aggressive boys can be daunting.

Eleven-year-old Aidan was demonstrating a range of "nuisance" behaviors, including not contributing to family chores, hitting his six-year-old brother, and "talking smart" to his parents. Aidan's mother, Gwen, was concerned, but conceded that she didn't want to be the disciplinarian. "He's like my best friend. I tell him everything, even the problems between me and my husband," she said. When Aidan was suspended from school for fighting, Gwen was upset. She didn't like the idea of "babysitting" Aidan while he played at home all day. She suggested that her husband, Scott, a construction manager, take Aidan to work with him. "Maybe he'll learn about how hard we work to provide for him," she said. As it turned out, Aidan was thrilled with this "punishment." (When misbehaving kids are forced out of school, they are often getting exactly what they want!) Scott did his best to supervise Aidan, but on the second day of this experiment Aidan was caught messing with the gears on an expensive company truck.

> ■ ■ ■
>
> If your son's speech is escalating into aggression, draw his attention back to his emotional state: "Harrison, are you calling him a show-off because he won the race? He's cheering because he's happy he's fast, not because he beat you. I know you're disappointed that you weren't first, but if you call him names, people will notice you in a bad way and think you're a sore loser. If you say 'Congratulations,' they'll think you're a good sport."

They came in for a family session. Aidan was cocky and responded to the pressure of the situation by remarking on his father's own work problems, including some things Gwen had confided to him. As he spoke, he seemed to have no sense of the serious-ness of the occasion, con-cern for his father's obvious displeasure in his recital, or his mother's growing dis-comfort. "He just doesn't get it," his father fumed. "He has no idea when he's gone too far, no ability to pull it together. He pushes and pushes the limits, then gets angry and pouts when people get upset with him!" Aidan's commun-ication reflected how his anger emerged from poor awareness of how his com-ments affected others, as well as his difficulty detect-ing other people's feelings.

Helping boys like Aidan means defining choices in situations they find emotionally confusing. Compre-hending the impact of their choices enhances their insight and ability to make good decisions. This heightens what psychologists call *executive awareness*, a person's ability to maximize his or her potential for judgment, self-control, and good decision making, a subject ad-dressed further in the next chapter.

> ■ ■ ■
>
> ### A Word in Time . . .
>
> For boys with poor awareness about how their comments affect others, parents can help by issuing warnings or offering alternative verbiage, such as:
>
> - "Your words are about to get you into trouble. When you say _____, people think _____."
> - "I'm feeling frustrated because I'm trying to tell you something and you keep interrupting me. Please wait until I let you know that I'm done talking, and then I'll listen to all your questions."
> - "Instead of saying, 'You're wrong!' to me, say, 'I disagree because . . .' "

Does Your Son Feel Uncomfortable Anywhere But the Top?

Aidan lacked awareness of emotion—his own and others—but he also lacked respect for the natural hierarchies in life, the principal one being that parents are superior to a child when it comes to au-thority. *Natural hierarchies* shape virtually all the groups we belong to and most activities in which we participate, and they help us under-stand our role in a particular context. For example, at school boys must not only grasp, but also respect, the authority of teachers and school personnel. The same requirements apply to getting along with a babysitter, boss, coach, bus driver, police officer, and, of course, parents. If, like Aidan, your son pushes the limits and then gets angry when the people he pushes get upset, the root of the problem may be his resistance to natural hierarchies.

For some boys, their resistance is obvious and plainspoken ("I'm not telling you anything—shut up!"). Other boys disguise their resistance to authority through more passive–aggressive tactics: the boy who continues to instigate "jokes" and disrupt a classroom despite redirection, who "forgets" to deliver important messages, or who shuts down a group's enthusiasm with negative comments: "If you guys want to go camping with our great scout leader, don't let me stop you."

The same boys might speak more pleasantly when initiating a conversation, speaking to a younger child or doting grandparent, or explaining something in their areas of "expertise." The trigger for these boys is that they cannot accept a socially subordinate position, and they use their words to demonstrate their defiance of social hierarchies.

Because many boys have such a strong will to mastery and authority, acknowledging natural hierarchies does not always come easily. Quite frankly, it is emotionally difficult to accept a rule or convention that feels like a violation of personal freedom. Although most adults can readily recognize the necessity and value of hierarchies, the strong-headedness of many boys causes them to struggle mightily with "authority issues." Although I wholeheartedly respect and support a boy's right to question authority in an appropriate way, none of us can afford to question all forms of authority, all the time, and expect to be successful socially. There's a difference between an opinionated boy who challenges authority while pushing the envelope in his role as editor of the school newspaper and a boy who uses profanity to verbally abuse his teacher. The editor may experience some conflict for his criticism of a school policy, but he's also learning the limits of his authority within a social system. In using the school paper as a vehicle for his opposition, he's entering into a dialogue and acknowledging an appropriate forum for dissenting speech. The boy who glibly swears at his teacher is on a one-way road to rejection, destined to learn mostly about personal failings.

Acceptance of Natural Hierarchies Starts with Family Solidarity

Families are where boys begin to learn about life's natural hierarchies. Before we can send boys into the world, where they will be expected to accept increasingly complex relationships and levels of authority, we must help them accept the natural laws that govern parent–child relationships. When we do this thoughtfully and with love, those laws are not a burden but a source of enduring emotional safety.

Gwen and Scott, Aidan's parents, hadn't instilled respect for natural hierarchies in their son because they didn't present a united front of authority. Similarly, Anthony and Patricia argue about how to raise their nine-year-old son, Owen. Anthony is an artist and wants Owen to have a childhood filled with expression, exploration, and self-determination. When Owen speaks in a disrespectful manner, Anthony says "He's going to learn that he's making a bad choice, but it's got to be *his* lesson to learn." Patricia is an attorney and wants him to have a consistent schedule, clear behavioral expectations, and regular chores. "I can't tolerate a sassy kid," says Patricia. "That's not the way I was raised." Anthony does the majority of the child rearing during the week, but on weekends the house becomes a battleground of conflicting instructions. Owen's frustration with this situation was evident in his increasingly surly communication. His parents complained about his frequent demands and inflexibility. Anthony and Patricia hammered out some rules for living and acceptable forms of communication that they both could agree on. For example, it would be okay for Owen to have a messy room if it was cleaned up by the weekend, and he was allowed to "argue" with parental decisions if he could provide solid reasons and spoke politely. Patricia said, "I wasn't happy about compromising my standards, but once Owen responded by relaxing his tone and being more patient while listening, the other stuff didn't bother me so much. Before, I'd look at his messy room and in my mind I'd hear him saying, 'You can't make me!' Now I feel like we're at a level of communication where I don't automatically react to him with anger. It gives me enough space to stop and consider what I really think about what he's saying. And now that the rules are clear, everything's not a negotiation. Owen is much calmer."

Boys with temperaments that veer toward anger have an especially high need for a family structure that emphasizes the parameters of acceptable behavior. Within this framework, you can clarify and show by example standards for positive family communication. *Although boys may express resistance toward externally imposed rules, clarity is at the core of emotional security.*

Autonomy versus Mutuality

Being driven by a strong need for autonomy can compromise a boy's flexibility and reasoning skills. He will likely be much more comfortable communicating in highly assertive ways that express his confidence in himself and his commitment to independence. Of course, this behavior is a normal part of growing up when it occurs occasionally, but some boys who communicate aggressively do so because they are intent on claiming the power of independence. Eight-year-old Trevor was fond of climbing to the top of rocks in his back-yard and proclaiming himself "King of the Mountain." Other boys would attempt to dethrone Trevor, only to discover that his will to be "king" infused him with great strength and an ability to hold his position. Trevor's parents marveled at his ability to ascend to the top of the rocks but also worried about Trevor's angry communication style during the game—"Get down, stupid!"—as well as how he carried this anger into his relationships with friends and siblings once the game was over.

"That game is a like a metaphor for his personality," his father said. "But he's the same in every situation. We went on vacation and stayed at a hotel with a pool. There was a group of kids there, but this time Trevor was the youngest. He kept challenging the other boys to races and contests even though he couldn't compete. They were nice enough kids, but they got sick of him. Everything was 'Cheater! I'll show you! Bet you can't do this! Hey you!' But we couldn't keep him out of that pool."

Trevor's mother added, "His brothers both made friends. But he didn't. I felt so bad for him, because his voice got very shrill, and everything was so stressful for him. He just couldn't deal with being the smaller one."

You probably shouldn't worry if you have a four-year-old who asserts, "I'm superboy, and I can smash the world!" But you should be somewhat concerned if you have a son like Trevor, a boy who has difficulty separating games from reality. Mutuality, which is at the heart of relationships, may be perceived as a threat to the control that so many boys covet and a disruption to the compelling fantasy of being an independent dominator. So boys like Trevor may end up missing out on friendships—and the social skills developed within them.

Keeping Games and Competition in Perspective

For most boys, games are where they explore the drama of life, including fantasies of winning and domination. Although this is a rite of passage for boys, taken to an extreme, such play can heighten self-consciousness and promote unrealistic feelings of invulnerability. Some boys with intensely competitive natures almost have a toxic reaction to playing games, which invariably leads to hurt feelings, name calling, or sulky quitting. They are generally unpleasant winners as well, crowing over their victory and "rubbing it in" to the losers. While it's difficult for almost all young boys to learn to play fairly and accept losses, by the time boys are in the second or third grade they should have made some strides in being able to handle the emotional challenges of mild competition. If Trevor reminds you of your own son, you can take measures like the following to downplay the competitive bent that may isolate him and to encourage mutuality.

- Play more collaborative games, such as Cranium, Cadoo, The Ungame, or Go, in which unequally skilled players can compete.
- Play games like checkers and chess, which can help boys with impulsivity and executive awareness problems because they emphasize sequential thinking and planning skills.
- Don't assume because boys are playing a "game" that it means fun—monitor their behavior and if things get out of control, put the game away.
- Teach your son to be a good winner and loser by giving him the appropriate words to say. "A winner doesn't show off; he thanks his competitors. A loser doesn't storm off; he congratulates the winner."
- If the fantasy component of a game seems to fuel unhealthy emotional responses in your son's daily life, limit his exposure.
- If you play games with your son, don't let him always win to avoid conflict. By the same token, handicapping to give him a fair opportunity to win occasionally will keep the game engag-

ing. Model appropriate speech, use humor, and help him become alert to his emotional responses.

It's Lonely at the Top

If you have any doubt about the truth of this statement, ask Peter. A contractor, Peter was very upset because his ex-wife was using his stint in juvenile detention as an adolescent, twenty years ago, as evidence against him in a bitter custody battle. "I have been a rebel my whole life. I can't help it, I hate to have anyone tell me what to do. That's why I had to have my own business, because I want to run things. I build great houses. I was chairman of a community housing group that basically did nothing for years, maybe built ten low-income units a year. Last year they completed seventy units. That was because of me, but they didn't appreciate it. They wanted team meetings and sweet talk, but I did what I had to do to get things done. When people give me 'advice,' I have to assume they don't respect me." Peter's lifelong commitment to pure autonomy had jeopardized his freedom, ruined his marriage, alienated colleagues, and hurt his children. Although Peter's fiery temperament was a part of who he was, he had never accepted responsibility for working with the behavioral liabilities that grew from that part of his personality. Peter needed to learn that he could express his autonomy in verbally constructive ways, which could earn him respect rather than alienation. When those pathways began to emerge in the course of therapy, he said to me, "Ever since I was a kid, I assumed I had to take respect if I wanted it. I never thought about what I lost in the process."

Sometimes boys are burdened with a temperament that makes it difficult for them to adjust to the conventions and expectations that govern community life. One way to understand the behavior problems that may accompany boys' anger is as a kind of revolt against the constraints society imposes on their desire for self-rule. Boys with angry temperaments seem to be wary of threats to their autonomy from an early age and are quick to act out in rebellion. At times their resentment of social demands is expressed through oppositionality and defiance. It's as though they're being dragged forcefully through the process of socialization and are intent on protesting the injustice of relinquishing their instinct for absolute freedom. Boys who are intent on self-rule inevitably clash with the hierarchies of family and communal life, which more often than not emphasize the needs of the group over those of the individual.

Boys who have a strong desire for respect and who tend to view interpersonal exchanges as zero-sum equations ("We can't both win") are a true challenge for parents. You must balance their need for respect and acknowledgment without fueling unwarranted feelings of self-importance or falling into habits of appeasement. Preemptive comments ("Our conversation is starting to take a wrong turn"), humor ("I'll admit you're a powerful ninja if you'll admit you look silly in those orange pants"), clarity ("I'd respect you more if you had lost the money and told the truth"), and redirection ("Why don't you ask me another way?") are some of the tools you'll need to help your son avoid experiencing the same losses that Peter did.

Is Your Son Trying to Hide His Vulnerability?

Anger is often a sham, hiding a terror of loss of self. Your son's anger may be driven by his anxious pursuit of total independence, as we've discussed. And behind that pursuit of autonomy may lie a crushing sense of vulnerability. When we try to encourage mutuality, our good intentions may be interpreted as a boundary violation or as an attempt to take unfair advantage of an element of vulnerability within boys. Carrie, a thirty-five-year-old teacher and mother of three boys, told me about her middle son, Marco. "He's always been tough. As a baby he'd have screaming fits, and when he was a toddler he'd get very frustrated when he saw his older brother doing something he couldn't do. He walked by ten months, and I think it was because he just had to keep up—he has a real competitive drive. When Marco's little brother was born, he was quite jealous. I remember rocking the baby one day and Marco came in the room and saw us. My husband was there, so I asked him to take the baby and then asked Marco, who was four at the time, if he wouldn't like to rock with me. He started to climb into my lap, but then I looked in his eyes and smiled. Something about that moment was too much for him. He said, 'I'm not going to rock. I'm not a stupid baby anymore,' and stormed off. I think he really wanted to be held and rocked, but it somehow felt humiliating to him too." Marco's reaction to his mother's offer illustrates how self-conscious boys can be when it comes to sharing affection. Although a boy's need for affection can be very strong, he may be extraordinarily self-conscious about showing it and may feel particularly vulnerable when he senses someone can read his mind before he's ready to have his feelings known.

Parents can help boys who feel ashamed about their softer emotions and who fear dependence by going slowly and helping them save face. While it may be a temptation, after finally getting a sweet word or well-deserved hug, to hammer the point home and teasingly say, "See, that wasn't so bad," your son may initially need you to accept his affectionate gestures in a more matter-of-fact manner.

And over the long term, keep in mind that boys who have a strong sense of themselves don't have to put up such a battle defending these boundaries. You'll find lots of ideas for helping your son develop a strong self-identity in Chapter 9.

Does Anger Make Your Son Feel Strong?

Help me with an experiment. Actually, this experiment is the psychoanalytic technique called *free association*. I'll give you a word—let's use *anger*—and you tell me all the other words you can think of that you associate with it. I'm going to guess that you might have thought of words like *mad, rage, fury, upset, mean, hurt, animosity, wrath, aggravation, exasperation, hostility,* or *annoyed.* This is a reasonable and good list, but it excludes one of the most important psychological associations with anger made by many boys. When words are in short supply, anger equals *strength.*

Before they're old enough to have any real power or status, boys learn to simulate authority through anger. Their ability to summon and portray anger can be seen in the "war of wills" with parents and peers alike. Anger is both the offensive and defensive weapon of choice when boys sense the pressure of socialization at the boundaries of their private selves. By showing us how angry they can become, they defy us to enter their personal space and declare their resistance to entering ours. If we are to help these boys across the communication divide, we will need to meet their resistance with determination and compassion. We will need to understand that anger is the default for a boy who feels caught between a world that demands social compliance and the voice within his own mind that insists on autonomy.

Socially resistant boys have an extraordinary knack for making well-meaning questions seem irrelevant, even foolish. I know of no other group of boys more eager to convince parents or therapists that they are "unhelpable." If we are too hasty in attempting to disarm their anger or resistance, these boys may feel as though we are trying to usurp their "strength."

The earlier we get started with helping boys find alternative paths to strength, the better chance they will have to build self-esteem based on real social accomplishment, rather than domination or intimidation. When we're confronted with our sons' anger, our persistence in acknowledging those feelings may be one of our best weapons in waging the battle for a meaningful relationship. Even if your son doesn't immediately reciprocate this acknowledgment, a parent's concern lives within his mind as an important source of support and self-esteem.

Is Anger a Shield That Conceals Your Son from Others?

While anger can be used to ward off vulnerability, it's also a disguise that many boys use to avoid revealing themselves to others. Boys can use anger to intimidate parents or peers, deflecting their questions and avoiding discussions of the things that really matter. Even the most experienced parents may back off from boys with angry dispositions, just because it can be so unpleasant to deal with that anger. It's important to remember that the ability to block inquiry is often a measure of a boy's sense of autonomy and power. So when he tries to keep you at a distance by using a certain tone, or avoiding eye contact, or in some way being resistant in an angry manner, recognize that he may feel he is competing with you for where the boundaries of privacy will be established.

Naturally, these boundaries change. For a seventeen-year-old boy not to want to discuss his girlfriend with his mother is not a totally unnatural phenomenon. However, a nine-year-old boy unwilling to discuss a conflict with his teacher should raise more concern. As parents, we're required to reassess our sons' boundaries throughout their lives, gauging when we should inquire and when we should give them some space. One way we can proceed is to simply teach our sons how to say they'd like some privacy or time to think things over, without reverting to anger or sullen withdrawal. If we can show that we'll respect their requests, we remove the need for them to hide behind a blustering façade. (We can also set some ground rules for issues, such as the health, safety, and whereabouts of our sons, that must remain open to discussion!)

■ ■ ■

Sometimes anger is the default emotion when more measured responses seem too complicated. Rather than letting his parents know that he's both proud and embarrassed that his voice is changing, and unwilling to ask them "not to notice" when his voice breaks, Todd avoids speaking and shuts down conversations with terse answers. At fifteen, Mohammed isn't sure he likes his new school and worries about taking the wrong bus transfer to get there, so he's sarcastic and scowling. Blake has a crush on a girl, and the thought of his parents plying him with interested advice and sex education is too humiliating. Could your son be using angry communication to avoid disclosing uncertainty about changes in his life?

Could the Real Message Be Depression?

Angry communication sometimes emerges in response to highly stressful situations that don't allow time for contemplation. Something that you find relatively benign may feel highly stressful to your son. A boy who wants to present the appearance of being sure of himself, who has difficulty reading the intentions of others, has a diffuse understanding of his own emotions, or lives in terror of embarrassment is at high risk of "overreacting." When boys are presented with a perceived threat to their autonomy or pride, they may reflexively react with anger, ready to compete and battle if they sense they have a chance of winning. Often this reflex doesn't take into account the long-term consequences of such a way of expressing themselves and doesn't even consider whether fighting is something worth doing.

This is partly a matter of temperament. Some boys, even from a young age, have "touchy" personalities. Even boys who once seemed shy and withdrawn can find their frustration turning to anger by the intrusion of other people into their personal psychological space. Sometimes the combination of adolescent hormones and increased size is enough to tip the balance and turn a withdrawn boy into a more antagonistic teenager. You may be able to draw some parallels from your son's early disposition to his current behavior. However, if your sunny, mild-tempered child has *suddenly* turned into a hostile alien, you might want to rule out depression, a changing personal situation (being bullied at school, a breakup), and drug abuse as possible causes.

When moodiness occurs without a precipitating event (and boys won't often tell you if there is one), it can be a challenge to determine whether this is just a tendency in a boy's temperament, a normal period of adolescent introversion, or a sign of a more serious mood problem developing. You may want to seek professional assistance to make this determination.

▪ ▪ ▪

Is He Mad or Sad?

Sometimes parents don't teach their sons how to describe a low or depressed mood in the misguided hope that this will somehow inoculate him against such feelings. Lacking another option, these boys then express sadness, loss, or guilt as anger. Boys often find it easier or more socially acceptable to show they're angry rather than sad. But in doing so, they miss opportunities for connection and healing.

Help Him Find the Words:
The Key to Transforming Your Son's Anger

Although angry and resistant boys often prompt strong negative feelings in adults, we can't lose sight of the fact that they have an emotional problem. They have no less emotion than other people but are often simply less capable of articulating their feelings. We have to help them find the words they need.

Suppose your kindergarten-age son is having trouble fitting together some Tinker Toys, and getting mad, starts throwing them against the wall. Encourage him to "use your words!" If he can't tell you what's upsetting him, offer suggestions: "Are you frustrated because that toy is hard to work? Can we think of a way together? If I give you a hint, you'll know how to do it all by yourself, and then you'll feel proud!" If he persists in acting out, take the toy away, gently explaining, "I don't understand what the problem is with this toy. When you can tell me what's wrong, we'll work together on fixing it." You've identified his emotion for him (frustration) and offered a solution that involves *working together, reinforcing the pleasure and satisfaction of reciprocal communication.* You've provided a consequence (removal of toy) that gives him an incentive to behave differently, a sure-fire way to demonstrate that his anger is ineffective. To motivate him further, amply praise him if he tries to do as you ask. The same steps can be effective with older boys. We'll miss important opportunities to shape our sons' insights if we focus on implementing consequences without also pointing to the emotions that accompany difficult situations.

If your son seems to express things strongly only when he's angry, try helping him find words to strongly express other kinds of emotions as well. The physical experience of expressing something strongly is part of being human, and boys have as much need to feel the adrenaline rush of expressing strong emotions as anyone else. Our job as parents is to help them channel that need into balanced ways of expressing a range of feelings.

Passive–Aggressive Social Communication

Overtly aggressive boys may be active manipulators, using words as blunt weapons, while other angry boys have a more passive–aggressive disposition. Some boys mope and fuss; others complain and blame. Boys with passive–aggressive communication can be self-pitying ("Why do I always have to . . ?"), uninvolved ("So what?"), or self-centered ("It will be boring for me!"). They throw up roadblocks ("It won't work"; "I'll do it later!") and instill blame ("What do you care?").

Kris, a young teenager whose parents wondered if he was depressed, refused to participate in family life. He was quiet and grumpy, declined to show enthusiasm for any activities his parents suggested, and rarely liked what was served for meals. He barely acknowledged his sisters, "forgot" about his chores, and seemed not to hear his parents until they repeated themselves several times. Mostly he sat in his room and listened to music or watched television. Family life seemed to revolve around enticing Kris to "come out of his shell," "enjoy himself," or get involved in something. It seemed the harder they tried, the less effective his family was.

When I talked to Kris, it became apparent that he was highly aware of his power over the family. Instead of disinterest, his lack of participation was more of a mulish refusal to "go along with the program." Rather than being overtly angry, Kris was passively aggressive, refusing to allow his family to reach him.

"My mom is always making me these special meals she thinks I'll like," he said. "She doesn't know what I want."

"Do you tell her?" I asked.

He shrugged his shoulders. "I tell her everything's fine; she just won't let it go."

"Isn't that because she knows everything's not fine?" I asked.

"It's no big deal. She can just do whatever she wants."

"But isn't all her effort a lot of extra work for her?" I inquired.

Kris didn't answer. "Do you think she's trying to do something nice for you?" I continued.

Kris looked at me, as if sizing me up. "Yeah, but maybe I just don't know what I want," he quipped irritably.

Kris's parents decided to take an entirely different tack with him. While still treating him kindly, instead of preparing meals for him they insisted that he make his own meals and once a week make dinner for the family. Rather than continue his allowance, they let him earn tips for preparing and serving the meal. They took away his television until he signed up for and attended an activity of his choice. Dinnertime discussion focused on how Kris had been useful to his family or household; privileges were attached to performance. "At first he made peanut butter and jelly sandwiches for supper and was very sarcastic. I guess our tips reflected the menu and the civility of the waiter," chuckled his father. "I showed him how to operate the gas grill and made him follow a recipe. He made hamburgers and salad the next week." "Are you still following through?" I asked. "You bet," said his father, "I think Kris may have found his calling. He invented a recipe for a breakfast taco, and it's good! You know, at first the whole thing was awkward. But once we got him moving

■ ■ ■

Boys who express their hostility passively or manipulatively must be brought out of their state of self-absorption. To begin to reclaim your son, try:

- Actively structuring his time so that he accomplishes something of merit every day. Ideally, this should be something for his family and his community.
- Clearly explaining the kind of communication that is and isn't acceptable.
- Linking privileges with positive communication.

Don't continue to reward bad behavior (including poor communication) with status quo, "life as normal" perquisites. Does your son still get an allowance, have the keys to the car, get to watch videos? Don't be afraid to take the heat in the short term for long-term gains.

and started refusing to accept his negative talk, he started to feel better."

For Kris, his parent's insistence that he accomplish something useful every day and focus his energy and attention outward provided important steps toward rehabilitating his self-esteem and interest in life. Boys who express their hostility passively or manipulatively must be brought out of their state of self-absorption. Work justifies feelings of self-worth. Boys who fraudulently inflate their importance without accomplishments to support this vision of themselves tend to either retreat or attack any encroachment, for fear that their deception will be revealed. When we help boys build a sense of real achievement, we make it safer for them to take down the walls of anger that surround them.

Resistance as Power

Some of the most challenging boys with whom I've worked used silence as a deviant expression of power. Leveraging this kind of power is especially important for boys who feel they have inadequate control over their lives. Parents often feel frustrated and impotent as words of all kinds—inquiry, concern, encouragement, support—seem to bounce off these boys and their well-rehearsed indifference. Discussions are often one-sided. Thoughts and unanswered questions are left hanging in the air. Unless you're well prepared for the challenges of these boys, you can end up "catching" the same alienation and despair that underlies their silence and social isolation.

Joseph's parents requested, pleaded, and finally demanded that he respond to their very great concerns about his bad grades and near total lack of effort in school. Over and over, they asked him to consider the consequences of failing a year of high school, and still he was unresponsive. His expression remained the same, and he spoke only when asked questions that could be answered in the simplest way. Joseph was content to let his parents cast frantic verbal nets as he leaned back in his chair, averting his eyes, determined not to give any sign that he was affected by the concern around him.

Joseph agreed to accept professional help, but was poorly equipped for an experience like counseling, which relies heavily on language. He could talk about his interest in Japanese animation, but couldn't articulate what he liked about it. He had very little descriptive language overall, rarely using adjectives. Discussions with Joseph worked best when

■ ■ ■

When boys use silence as a passive–aggressive weapon, shake up the routine and try relationship-building activities that will reopen the lines of communication.

- Develop a weekend ritual or project. Mario had his son, Jorge, help him clear a path through their thick woods in return for car privileges. Persisting despite Jorge's initial muttering and foot dragging, in a few weeks they'd come home filthy, scratched . . . and talking.
- Learn something new together. A complex task, such as rebuilding an engine or learning to sail, requires functional speech ("Hand me that wrench") and problem solving ("Should we reef the sail?") that can develop into more relational communication ("We did a good job today . . . ").
- Find a common social goal. Volunteer, attend a rally, or protest together.
- Provide opportunity for accomplishment.

they came from a concrete reference point—almost like show-and-tell. Attempts to get Joseph to talk about himself were met with stiffened resistance and even less engagement in therapy.

When you reach this type of social and communicative stalemate with a boy, you need to rethink your entire approach. What are his primary needs? So often as parents we react strongly to something like failing grades without appreciating the more fundamental issues underlying that problem. We may have lost touch with our sons. The diverse influences that flow through a boy's mind can cause him to drift, making it difficult to "reach him" the way you could when he was younger. When we are trying to reach boys who resist us in a passive–aggressive way, sometimes we need to reduce their autonomy and reclaim them as our own! By rolling up our sleeves and getting involved in their day-to-day activities, we can help them forge a path out of their attitudinal rut. Our participation in problem solving teaches boys an important lesson about the value of collaboration.

Antisocial Boys

When boys become self-absorbed and antisocial, compliance with social expectations may be viewed as a sign of weakness. What these boys prefer is a system in which they can learn the rules for competition and assert themselves, often through physical means, as a governing figure in a particular social group.

Underdeveloped Empathy

Boys indifferent or opposed to social communication rarely seek cooperation and reciprocity. They often view people as "instruments of use" who can be manipulated. Some boys can impress us as so alienated that expecting them to initiate social or emotive communication feels unrealistic. But this may come back to words—or the lack of them. In a recent study led by psychologist Bryan Loney, published in the *Journal of Clinical Child and Adolescent Psychology,* antisocial boys with "callous-unemotional" dispositions were found to have a delayed cognitive response to words that describe emotions. (This was in contrast to more impulsive types of antisocial boys, who tended to respond to emotive words at much faster rates.) The study did not reveal whether their alienation from emotion words stemmed from these boys' innate callous disposition or a lack of exposure to feeling words contributed to their stunted emotional development. So we can't say that boys become antisocial when their emotional literacy hasn't been cultivated. But I believe exposing them early and intensively to the language of emotions, and modeling positive social behavior, can at least set them on the right path toward social interest.

The Surprising Status of Being Antisocial

In school, angry or antisocial boys can be found in both small groups dedicated to an "outsider" attitude toward school and peers, and larger groups made up primarily of average kids. Because these boys are often quick to assert social control, they can command the attention of peers, sometimes winning peer approval through expressions of bravado. Few things are so compelling to middle school boys as one among them who seems to be able to "outsmart" a teacher or school administrator. They also rule because they are not inhibited from hurting or humiliating challengers. As a result, antisocial kids may themselves have an elevated status, unfortunately being positively reinforced for those qualities that are their ultimate undoing.

A study led by psychologist Phillip Rodkin at Duke University examined both popular-prosocial and popular-antisocial fourth- to sixth-grade boys. Although those in the latter group were identified as "tough" by peers, as well as themselves, this group had other attributes, including physical competence, that supported a strong level of social connection with peers. Whatever concerns one might have about the quality and consequences of these social connections, it's clear

> ■ ■ ■
>
> Research findings indicate that contrary to what might be expected, younger antisocial children might be well regarded by peers ("popular") and have good self-esteem. However, as children grow older, aggression that once was tolerated becomes a social liability.

that aggressive boys can be well regarded by peers and also feel satisfied with their self-image, including hurtful communication, at least in some respects. The problem with concluding that aggression isn't so bad is that as antisocially inclined boys get older, aggression escalates accordingly, eventually leading to social rejection and alienation. What fourth-grade boys find amusing loses its luster as children make the transition to adolescence and the emergence of more mature social sensibilities.

Meghan, the mother of a sixteen-year-old, told me this: "My son was very popular through elementary school and junior high. It wasn't until he went to high school that things changed for him. There

> ■ ■ ■
>
> If your son is being rewarded by his peers for less-than-admirable behavior (teasing, name calling), try these ideas:
>
> - Provide negative consequences for the behaviors (parental disappointment, loss of privileges, public apology, and the like).
> - Support his teacher in developing strategies to handle the situation in school.
> - Help him convert his "social capital" into more positive forms of leadership.
> - Discuss the short- and long-term consequences for him and his "targets."
> - Teach him how to speak powerfully and persuasively without hurting others.

were some kids from his old schools there, but instead of being friends, they froze him out. When he was younger he wasn't always as sensitive to some other kids as he should have been. But they never gave him a chance to make it up to them."

The Self-Absorption of Antisocial Boys

While shy boys may be involved in their individual pursuits because they feel socially self-conscious and are seeking the kind of mastery that can be found within their individual challenges, the self-absorption of antisocial boys has much more to do with being self-centered. This seems to speak to these boys' difficulty with sharing themselves with other people. Antisocial boys may be consumed with their own status and their own need to assert themselves within a group. They can become so intent on this need that they limit their capacity for empathy, deliberately shutting down their feelings for others.

Some antisocial boys remain loners, preferring to stay on the periphery of any type of social interaction. When they can be engaged, adults may find them intelligent and reasonably articulate. However, these boys often have a strong aversion to expressing themselves because they associate open communication with a type of emotional vulnerability they find repulsive.

Terry, an eighteen-year-old with no overt behavioral problems, is a good example. He's never been in trouble. He is highly intelligent and has started his own Internet business selling rare coins. Terry's parents confide that they worry that he "is not normal." He has no friends and is obsessed with making money. He lives within the family like an outsider. "When he goes to his room, it's like he's walking through the lobby of a hotel and I'm the desk clerk. He doesn't talk to me except to ask for messages," said his mom. "He has almost no interest in the rest of the family," complained his father.

I asked when Terry's parents first became worried. They said that as a child Terry had insisted on winning games and was unusually focused on "getting his fair share." When he was ten, he started selling goldfish to relatives and neighbors. After a while, the novelty wore off and nobody wanted to buy any more fish. "We thought he was hurt. But Terry just flushed all the extra goldfish down the toilet and said, 'I know other things to sell.' " That's when he got into old coins. By eighth grade, Terry was spending most of his spare time at a flea market where he'd started his coin business. When his parents tried to encourage him to attend social events or make friends, he'd say, "I'm fine, leave me alone." His father said, "For years we let it go, thinking he would grow out of it, learn to relate to the other kids more. It's just gotten worse. He recently refused to come on vacation with us because of his business. He always has a logical reason to avoid getting involved."

Boys like Terry require parental intervention at an early age. You cannot expect to change all aspects of a boy's personality, but it's reasonable to believe you can introduce more balance. The social resistance of boys like Terry needs to be met with firm guidance about the value of things beyond the boundary of themselves. Terry's parents missed opportunities to encourage his development, because they didn't counteract his social resistance with some form of social *insistence*—insistence that he become more of a participant in family and community life and that he expand his range of personal satisfaction beyond such narrow interests.

Probing the Mind–Body Connection

Interestingly, antisocial boys have a strong propensity for demonstrating a particular physiological characteristic, highly predictive of their antisocial dispositions. In a 2004 study published in the *Journal of the American Academy of Child and Adolescent Psychiatry,* Jame Ortiz and Adrian Raine reported the results of a meta-analysis relating heart rate to antisocial behavior. Individuals who demonstrate antisocial behavior are more likely to have lower heart rates. Further, the

■ ■ ■

"I'm Fine, Leave Me Alone"

Boys who tend to be self-absorbed or who ward off attempts at connection with others benefit from early intervention, when it's easier to develop social interest. By the time they reach adolescence, it can be hard to sell them on the pros of socialization, because you'll have less influence on how that socialization takes place and less opportunity to build social skills incrementally. If you have an older boy who tunes the world out and rejects involvement with others, he may benefit from working with you, an adult mentor, or a therapist who can strategically guide his social development.

study suggests that the relationship between physiology and personality may also explain the higher prevalence of antisocial behavior among males, since there are "robust gender differences in resting heart rate, with males' being lower than females'." Surprisingly, the gender differences in heart rate have been reported to be in place by three years of age!

The Ortiz and Raine study suggests that for psychological interventions to be effective with antisocial children, they must have the effect of elevating heart rate. Extrapolating from the study's data and conclusions, we can see that many of the traits exhibited by some boys of few words, including low verbal output and social inactivity, might also be expressions of a physiological disposition toward low emotional arousal. Many therapists would likely agree with Ortiz and Raine's suggestion to provide interventions that elevate heart rate, effectively raising emotional arousal and attention. Mental health professionals have long known that a moderate degree of excitement enhances learning. However, I suspect that anyone who has worked with this difficult group of boys can identify with how frustrating it is to get them psychologically (and, by extension, physiologically) engaged in therapy. It may also explain why the cliché of the tough-but-tender coach or army sergeant, who breaks through to the arrogant or out-of-control young man, may hold a grain of truth. These types of authority figures are experts at increasing heart rate!

■ ■ ■

When you want to get a resistant boy more engaged in communication, it may be helpful to start an activity that will cause a natural increase in heart rate. This may be one reason boys talk more easily after a vigorous game of basketball or after a run or some other type of sports. If your son is resisting communication, is not looking at you, and you feel the conversation is painfully slow or sparse, it's probably a cue that you need to do something to accelerate his thinking and responsivity. Get out of the chair, walk as you talk, challenge him to clear a jump or hit a target—anything to literally get things moving. Through these activities boys find it easier to be disclosing, because they are not feeling so directly confronted, and because physiologically they are being activated.

The Call to Be Wild

While we've been talking primarily about boys driven by self-absorption and a manipulative social disposition, closely related are boys who have a need for constant stimulation. These boys are thrill seekers, who impulsively engage in activities that may have devastating consequences for themselves or others. Through such behavior they often impact the lives of other people adversely, with little regard for consequences. A constant search for stimulation undermines the focus required for effective communication, and many of these boys have attention deficits that fuel their need for perpetual excitement. Although these boys' behavior often strays outside social conventions, their actions are typically driven by the thrill of risk taking rather than an absence of conscience, as might be the case for more seriously antisocial boys.

A friend recently told me about taking her toddler daughter to a local fast-food restaurant that had a play area where kids could climb through tunnels and go down slides. "I only take her at off times, because you see these wild boys there, around four or five years old, and they're yelling like crazy, and they'll climb right over your kid. They have no idea how they could hurt or scare a little one." I asked her how the boys' parents usually handled it, and she thought a moment. "You know, those are usually the weary parents who look burned out!"

Boys who get wildly involved in play, especially kinesthetic play, often can't put the brakes on. They grab toys, yell wildly, knock others down, throw rocks at animals, and instigate dangerous dares, not so much from malicious intent but from an addiction-like response to the sensation of motion and the thrill of the hunt. Their communication skills are often significantly underdeveloped from lack of practice. These boys need frequent intervention and coaching to assist with thinking through the consequences of their choices and actions. Encouraging this type of awareness is the necessary first step toward building their capacity for social consideration and communication.

Don't Back Away

Persistence is a key factor in working with the types of social communication challenges explored in this chapter. It's human nature to want to avoid angry people, yet if we remember that anger may be a boy's default rather than choice, perhaps we can learn to reframe what we see and hear in a way that heightens our empathy for our sons. Anger and resistance in boys are expressions of social difficulties that call for guidance and support, and although our sons can't tell us as much, they don't want us to back away.

SEVEN

Navigating the Challenges
of Learning and Attention Problems

■ ■ ■

When Palmer started school, the whole family felt turned upside down. Suddenly the quiet boy who had been his parents' pride and joy was having trouble making friends, and his teacher reported that he had a negative attitude and was underachieving academically. At first his parents, Mona and Don, thought it was because he was having a hard time making the transition from being at home, where, said Mona, "he always had my undivided attention and support. I thought when he didn't talk so much he was just being like his dad, who also tends to be on the quiet side, but always thinking."

Once they had a chance to see that the teacher wasn't exaggerating, Palmer's worried parents had him evaluated and eventually enrolled him in a school for kids with learning disabilities, where the teachers started helping them find Palmer's strengths and understand his challenges. It turned out that Palmer had dyslexia, along with problems with distractedness. His reading started improving, but his parents weren't sure whether his inattention contributed to his reading problems or vice versa. They also found that Palmer was at least a little obsessive–compulsive—he hated it when the "rules" changed, and transitions were the hardest times for him.

But the biggest surprise to Don and Mona was how many social problems Palmer had along with his learning and attention problems. It was as though when his reading development stalled, so did his social skills. Palmer seemed less confident around peers and became noticeably quieter as a result. When he did join conversations, he often spoke too fast or talked over other children. Palmer just wasn't on the same page with other kids.

When Cory began to have problems with distraction and hyperactivity at age six, his parents moved quickly to get him help, and he was diagnosed with attention-deficit/hyperactivity disorder (ADHD). After Cory started on medication and began seeing a school counselor, they saw improvement in his ability to learn and to follow school rules. "It was a huge relief," related Cory's mother. "We were concerned because Cory had been bringing home a note about his disruptive behavior almost every day, and we were worried that sooner or later he would give up on school." Fortunately, intervention helped Cory get through elementary school with much less difficulty. In fact, Cory's improvement had become so routine that his parents assumed that transition to middle school would simply be the next step. But when Cory made the leap to the social demands of seventh grade, he found himself struggling with what I sometimes call the "rules of engagement."

In essence, Cory felt awkward about approaching other students, even kids he knew from elementary school. Although his medicine reduced his hyperactivity and he had learned some behavioral strategies for "putting the brakes on," relatively little attention had been given to the social dimensions of Cory's ADHD. As for many kids with ADHD, the social impact had not really been noticeable until Cory reached middle school. Now he and his peers were expected to be more independent. Students had more freedom during unstructured time, and there was more socializing after school. Cory's father commented, "He seems kind of out of it to us, like he's confused by how older kids talk and relate to each other. We thought we had this ADHD problem taken care of, but what he's going through now—I don't think medication is going to be the answer."

Leon, a twelve-year-old with a nonverbal learning disability, had received intensive help with math difficulties in school. His parents appreciated his hard work in math but were concerned that socially he seemed so distant and inhibited. His mother was perplexed about how a boy so insightful about practical matters could be so confused by personal situations or experiences. "The other day I was in a terrible mood from work," his mother explained. "I came home very upset, and I knew he could see that, but he never said anything to me. And this kind of thing has happened before. We'll be at the mall or visiting friends, and everybody will be impressed by something that Leon says. But they don't see that he doesn't know how to take his insight to the next step. Why is it so difficult for him to show someone he cares when I know he really does?"

Some boys of few words have communicative and social challenges shaped by temperament or the emotional atmosphere of family life, as discussed in the two preceding chapters. But others have social and expressive difficulties connected with learning disabilities or attention deficits or, not infrequently, both. The ways in which these neuropsychological problems contribute to social difficulties are complex. The interventions designed to help boys overcome dyslexia or a nonverbal learning disorder, inattention, or hyperactivity pay little attention to boys' (or girls') social growth. It's not that the professionals providing treatment and implementing special accommodations at school don't care about this part of a child's development. It's just that time and funds are limited, and often the social issues are considered a lower priority.

I consider surmounting the social challenges that come with learning disorders and ADHD every bit as important as helping these boys learn to read, to pay attention in class, or to manage their behavior. We've discussed the long-term consequences of social communication challenges, and the solutions we devise should give due attention to the social learning needs of boys who are very young. While a lot of attention is given to how to intervene with teenagers, relatively little focus is placed on the learning and social dynamics that lead to adolescents developing the problems they have. Of course, we need to reach out to boys of all ages, but the optimal time to intervene in social development is when we first see learning and attention problems on the horizon. In this chapter I'll explain why. In the process, I'll help you see what you can do to help your son socially and expressively if he has an attention or learning problem— you may find yourself at the helm in working through these problems with your child. And if you're not sure whether your son has one of these problems, I hope the boys described in the following pages will give you some idea of whether such deficits could be at the root of your son's uncommunicative behavior and what actions you can take to find out more.

Seemingly simple things, like knowing how to introduce themselves, maintaining the flow of conversation, and taking turns, can be immensely difficult tasks for boys who don't readily perceive social communication or remember how to apply communication skills. Yet without such skills, boys with learning or attention problems may never gain the social competence they have the power to achieve, and their adult lives will be poorer for it.

As discussed in Chapter 1, there is considerable ongoing investigation into why boys

■ ■ ■

Boys are disproportionately affected by learning disorders and attention deficit problems. Approximately five boys are diagnosed for every girl.

are so much more vulnerable to learning and attention problems than girls. Whatever conclusions these studies yield, we'll undoubtedly continue to find that learning and attention problems are multidimensional. *A true appreciation of these challenges requires that we acknowledge the complexity of learning disabilities and ADHD and the unique, variable ways in which children are affected by these disorders.* If you suspect your son may have one of these problems, keep in mind that a good diagnostic evaluation (see Chapter 11) should consider the neuropsychological, emotional, environmental, and social factors impacting your child as they reflect his individuality and unique circumstances. To complicate matters, these syndromes also often interact with the personality and behavioral dynamics, such as aggression and withdrawal. So it's not always easy—for psychologists or parents—to fit boys into clearly defined categories. My goal here is to encourage you to consider whether a learning or attention problem may be part of the picture for your own boy of few words—and how you can help if you believe that's the case.

The vast majority of professionals working with children and adolescents diagnosed with learning disabilities, ADHD, or both recognize the impact of learning and attention problems on communication and social competence. In a large-scale research review that examined the social competence of children with learning disabilities, Dr. Elizabeth Nowicki compiled the results of thirty-two studies conducted on this subject since 1990 and found strong evidence that children with learning disabilities in mainstream classrooms are at "social risk" as compared with classmates without learning disabilities. She also found

■ ■ ■

Boys with learning problems that limit self-awareness may not notice their own social learning challenges. If your own observations of your son leave you concerned, don't let his assurances that "there's no problem" deter you from considering his difficulties carefully and perhaps talking to his teachers or other professionals to get another perspective.

that classmates much preferred other students without learning disabilities. Perhaps both a blessing and a concern, Nowicki's study noted that while youth with learning disabilities are aware of formal learning deficits, they are much less aware of their social difficulties. This finding is strongly corroborated by my own evaluations of boys with learning disabilities and ADHD, who frequently rate themselves as popular and socially well adjusted, despite teacher and parental reports to the contrary.

How Boys Learn to Communicate

To understand how communication difficulties are intertwined with learning and attention problems, you need to know something about the neuropsychological processes involved in learning. Of particular concern are certain aspects of auditory processing—how the brain makes sense of different sounds so that a person can understand and hear language. Social comprehension relies heavily on being able to receive language cues on multiple levels—what is being said, how it's being said, and why it's being said. A boy's ability to synthesize these different levels of understanding is the foundation of his confidence when it comes to social communication. As we'll see, listening is where communication skills begin.

The Sounds of Words

Many children with learning disabilities, particularly reading disorders, have a problem specifically with *phonological awareness*. This very valuable aspect of auditory processing involves being able to hear and remember word sounds and relate those sounds to written words. Phonological awareness is closely related to *phonemic awareness*, which has to do with being able to aurally discriminate the forty-four phonemes (the smallest units of word sounds) that make up the English language—for example, being able to clearly distinguish between the sound of "p" and "b" and to "hear" those sounds in your mind while reading those letters. These auditory processing skills are developmental hurdles that are typically achieved during preschool and early elementary grades. Although phonological awareness may improve even into the middle school years, language is learned best and most easily during its "critical period," usually thought to be before age eleven. It is during these years that the brain can most efficiently absorb and retain language learning.

> ▪ ▪ ▪
>
> *Phonological awareness* is a central auditory processing skill that enables a person to hear and remember word sounds and relate those sounds to written words. This skill allows the brain to decode words by breaking them down into smaller sound chunks called *phonemes*.

Angry That He Can't Keep Up

Five-year-old Royce was diagnosed with auditory processing difficulties in preschool, and the fact that these difficulties had delayed his learning of letters was presented as the primary reason for holding him back from starting kindergarten. But that wasn't his only problem. When Royce became frustrated that he wasn't learning as well as other children, he would engage in aggressive outbursts that prompted his teacher to say, "What he cannot clearly express he makes up for in volume," and that derailed the whole class—which is exactly what Royce wanted, albeit unconsciously.

In addition to affecting learning, difficulty with processing word sounds can have social consequences, as it did with Royce. It isn't until preschool that many boys first become aware of their learning differences, and that awareness may be anxiety provoking—if only on an unconscious level. The angry acting-out behavior of boys in this situation seems to reflect their strong will to assert themselves as having a "voice" despite their experiences of frustration and failure.

Phonological processing (hearing and remembering word sounds) is necessary for reading and verbal comprehension skills. In turn, these skills are important in developing social comprehension and interest. Think about all the interactions that occur in a normal conversation—the careful choice of some words, the nuanced inflection of others, the confirmation or contradiction of certain statements. A boy with poor phonological processing skills is more likely to misunderstand what he's hearing and be unable to convey his thoughts effectively. It's as if he were trying to converse in a second language that he's only partially familiar with—he might get his main point across, but his capacity to fully express himself would be limited. The person he'd be talking to could even get frustrated or talk louder—the way some people do when speaking to someone who doesn't understand because the language they are using isn't the listener's native language! After a while, he might conclude that conversing is tiresome or risky. Boys with poor phonological processing skills tend to "tune out" the discourse that builds and fortifies relationships. If this describes a boy you know, your support can encourage him to persevere with building the conversational skills that don't come "naturally."

Royce's parents were pleasantly surprised to discover that when he began speech–language therapy, his language learning skills improved and his frustration level decreased. My own work with Royce focused on helping him find more constructive ways to gain attention, although his pride made it difficult for him to talk to me about his learning challenges. This is an important consideration when working with many boys—it is a practical necessity to emphasize achievement. Rather than avoiding the critical issues, focusing on accomplishment means building an alliance of trust and positive regard. The alliance fuels a child's growth because it provides an emotionally safe context in which boys can look at themselves openly and honestly. Time spent building a strong partnership is a sound investment that consistently pays off.

> ■ ■ ■
>
> Helping boys with learning problems begins with a strong alliance forged through mutual respect and verbalizations of a boy's strengths: "Yes, you do need some extra help with reading, but don't forget that you're ahead in math." "I know you can't think of what to say all the time, but remember that time you explained about dinosaurs to Ellie—you were amazing." "Garth, I'll be with you every step of the way. Whenever you need help with homework, let me know. I believe you can succeed because you're one of the hardest workers I've ever known."

Royce's parents were right to have him evaluated by a therapist for speech and language problems. The earlier such problems are addressed, the more effective these interventions will be in helping boys develop verbal skills. The plasticity of a young boy's brain gives him a decided advantage in making use of such intervention. Just as we increase our chances of becoming a champion tennis player or concert pianist if we get lessons very early in life, a boy's reading and social abilities benefit most from early support of auditory processing skills.

Overall, the role of auditory processing is very significant for the boys we're talking about, because, anatomically speaking, males have brains that are less efficient than female's in processing language. While females use both hemispheres of their brains to process language, males rely primarily on the left hemisphere. As we discussed earlier, the part of the brain that spans the two hemispheres (corpus callosum) and facilitates communication between them is generally more bulbous and consequently more efficient for processing language in females. Fascination with the corpus callosum began in the early 1980s and has resulted in numerous experiments and research projects to investigate its impact on the communication differences between males and females. Although gender differences in the size and shape of the corpus callosum were first detected during autopsies, more recently neuroimaging technology has given scientists detailed pictures and new insights about this important part of the brain.

The effect of this gender difference is that while boys are struggling to learn language with a more limited part of their brains, some girls are accelerating and passing boys by being able to access a greater proportion of their cognitive resources for receptive and expressive language development. This may partially explain why girls are often six to twelve months ahead of boys in verbal learning by the time they reach elementary school. Of course, there are boys who are exceptions to this gender phenomenon, but boys of few words are notable examples of the unfortunate developmental discrepancy.

When first meeting a child whose parents or teachers are concerned about social skills deficits, therefore, I am always interested in the child's auditory processing skills. Sometimes a referral to an audiologist can be revealing and lead to the best possible help for a particular boy. Audiologists can screen for what is called a *central auditory processing disorder,* which can include deficits in phonological awareness. Many psychologists also screen for auditory processing deficits as part of a learning disability evaluation. (We'll talk more about how to use the professionals available to you in Chapter 11.)

Learning to Read and Reading to Learn

Auditory processing skills play a central role in your son's ability to learn, enjoy, and effectively use language. Of particular importance is that his ability to hear word sounds strongly predicts how easily he will develop reading skills. And, it turns out, the ability to read is critical to your son's achieving a number of social milestones.

In the past ten years, the study of learning disabilities has seen a remarkable revolution in the conceptualization of dyslexia. Dr. Sally Shaywitz and her colleagues at Yale University have used medical imaging technology to map brain activity during reading, leading to new insights about the neuropsychology of reading, including the cognitive "microskills" that make reading possible. Before such investigations revealed these mechanisms, those with reading problems were sometimes misunderstood as unmotivated or unintelligent. Because research underscores the importance of phonological processing, intervention for reading disabilities now emphasizes skills and drills designed to fortify phonological awareness. Essentially, these drills teach students to learn words phonetically, both as a form of reading remediation and, for younger children, as an important mode of *preventing* reading disorders.

What's significant to boys of few words, however, and may be somewhat surprising, is that phonological processing is also a critical element in social competence. Both reading and verbal comprehension contribute to your son's ability to relate to others socially. Learning disabilities research to date has not pinned down the exact connection between phonological skills and social competence, but it does indicate a significant overlap between learning skills and social adjustment. That is, those who demonstrate difficulty with reading skills also often show poor social adjustment.

Reading is incredibly important as a primary way our sons learn about how people relate socially, including the way people speak to one another and how they think through problems. Reading greatly expands their social and emotional vocabulary, as it does for all of us, and helps them visualize the diverse ways personal interactions can occur. Books draw boys into the psychological realm of different people's lives, allowing them to learn from the commonalities and variations of the characters and experiences portrayed. As our sons become more sophisticated readers, they can think and debate about the meaning of an author's depictions. Our sons' beliefs and insights are, in part, born from this inner dialogue.

> ■ ■ ■
> Psychologists have excellent tests for word–sound awareness and reading decoding skills, which measure overall level of comfort with language and how effectively a child or adolescent can express himself. Boys with phonological processing problems generally find reading difficult and as a result are below average in reading interest and comprehension.

The relatively slow pace of reading also allows narrative detail to be processed and integrated at a much deeper level than it is in watching a film about the same story. As writer and scholar C. S.

Lewis commented, "Literature adds to reality, it does not simply describe it. It enriches the necessary competencies that daily life requires and provides."

Reading is essential exercise for the mind—especially if you have a boy of few words at home. Although television and movies expose boys to all kinds of language, the visual and spoken components of those mediums limit the potential for imagination and the important psychological process of projection. Reading requires boys to construct realities that will inevitably be personal, perhaps even autobiographical, because those realities are formed from the unique experiences that make up each boy's life. Because the lives of so many boys have been touched by learning or attention problems, we might justifiably worry that when it comes to reading skills, boys are increasingly being divided into two groups, the haves and have-nots. Given the social liabilities of not being a reader, membership in the latter group is something to be avoided to the greatest extent possible.

Ironically, becoming a good reader, which is a solitary act, can even bolster a boy's social comprehension and interest. One young boy I worked with was able to relate vignettes from his Harry Potter books to some of the social dynamics in his class. His reading of the Harry Potter stories had become an interpretive lens through which he could make sense of his social world. For him, Harry Potter's courageous battles against evil, and how Harry's small band of friends helped him, provided him with an imaginative framework to deal with his own personal crisis, which was how peers at school responded to his stuttering.

■ ■ ■

If your son struggles with reading because of an auditory processing problem, it's critical that he get whatever assistance he needs in learning to read—not just for the sake of becoming literate and succeeding academically, but because reading will enhance the social skills that also may be weakened by his lack of phonological awareness.

Hearing Words:
The Yellow Brick Road to Social Communication

If you have a son who has a learning disability, or who you now suspect might, you can see why it's important to intervene assertively:

problems with auditory processing and other deficits that hamper reading and language skills can lead to a dead end for a boy's social competence. I'm not suggesting that every boy with a phonological awareness problem will end up unable to get along socially as an adult. I am suggesting, however, that such boys follow a complicated path. We can give boys of few words a much needed jump start toward social ease if we recognize their need for help with social communication skills as soon as a learning problem is suspected.

The diagram on the following page illustrates *one way* of thinking about how phonological awareness contributes to social and emotional development. It depicts my conviction that auditory processing skills constitute one important path to *prosocial* behavior and emotional literacy. Acting prosocially means your son is motivated to use his knowledge and skills to enhance relationships. The diagram illustrates nested levels of language skills and social ability, with the achievement of each new capability being supported by the skills built into previous levels. In other words, having good phonological awareness helps promote expressive language skills; with the right combination of ability, opportunity, and encouragement, expressive language will in turn help to foster social comprehension. However, successive levels of development are not necessarily guaranteed. A boy might develop social comprehension, correctly perceiving other people's thoughts and behavior, but for reasons related to environment and/or temperament not progress to using that social knowledge in a way that contributes to his social development. (Clinical psychologists are, unfortunately, all too familiar with adults who use social comprehension in a manipulative, antisocial manner.) *We shouldn't assume that poor phonological awareness will lead to antisocial behavior, but good listening skills help open the door to positive social progress.*

Although many educators and psychologists recognize that syndromes like dyslexia are frequently associated with social difficulties, there has been relatively little research that explains the mechanism of that connection. One exception is a study by a group of researchers, led by Dr. Tova Most, at Tel Aviv University. Dr. Most and colleagues examined the link between phonological awareness and social functioning among preschool children, hypothesizing that both tasks rely on similar cognitive skills. They found that children identified as being at high risk for the development of learning disabilities, due to poor phonological skills, had significant difficulty with peer relationships. These children tended to have lower levels of peer acceptance

FIGURE 7.1.
Being able to hear
word sounds . . .
builds social
communication and
emotional
development.

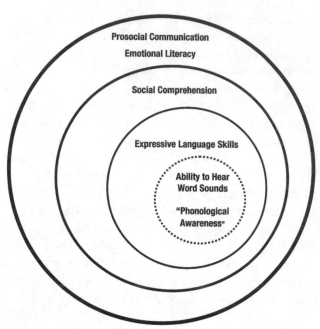

Prosocial Communication
Emotional Literacy

Social Comprehension

Expressive Language Skills

Ability to Hear
Word Sounds

"Phonological
Awareness"

than classmates and had far fewer friends. From an emotional perspective, children with phonological deficits perceived themselves as lonelier than peers and overall felt less confident. This study highlights the reciprocal nature of phonological processing and social skills. Auditory processing challenges begin shaping the way children are perceived by others almost as soon as they form their first significant social group (generally in preschool). Of concern is that Dr. Most's study also highlights how quickly children can become aware of their differences and encounter the social and emotional consequences of learning problems.

The neuropsychological problems that underlie deficits in reading and pho-

■ ■ ■

Research indicates that preschool children at risk for learning disabilities due to poor phonological awareness have more social difficulties, feel lonelier and less confident, and have fewer friends than their peers. If your child is having social problems in school, evaluation for an underlying learning disability may be warranted. In addition, you may wish to consider if, and how, preschool can provide appropriate care for your son.

nology are also associated with speech and articulation difficulties. Problems with speech development sometimes provide early clues about prospective learning and social challenges. Nate, a four-year-old with a cherubic smile and a head of red curls, had been born prematurely and experienced some speech delays. He had told his mother that "nobody plays with me" at day care, and in fact, when she observed him with other children she could see some differences. Most kids were busy chattering and interacting, but Nate was quiet; occasionally he'd sit near a group or silently offer a toy to a peer, but more often than not the other child would take it and go off and play with someone else. "Nobody was being mean to him, but it was like he was invisible. He just didn't have the communication skills to get in the flow of things. I think school was just too much for him to take on yet," Nate's mother said.

Ultimately, Nate's mother opted for an individual babysitter. She searched to find someone who would patiently engage him in conversation, to ease his anxiety about communication difficulties and spare him from the potentially harmful comparisons he was making between himself and peers. Of course, Nate will eventually have to go to school, but that transition will likely be much easier with the development of improved communication skills. His mother may not realize it, but making a relatively small adjustment in his early experience can provide exponentially positive results for Nate. Many, if not most, children do well in preschool. But by considering Nate's individual needs, his mother found a flexible, creative solution that worked better for *him*.

Next Stops:
Expressive Language Skills and Social Competence

Detection of meaning while listening to speech also supports the development of expressive language skills. Good auditory attention and processing allow children to begin hearing the way language is used and to extract meaning and suggestion from speech. As we've seen, boys are at a decided disadvantage as compared with girls when it comes to language processing and generally struggle more than girls when it comes to emotion detection. Scientists have hypothesized that this is because the brain's right hemisphere is primarily responsible for emotion detection, and the strong tendency of males is to rely on the left hemisphere for language processing. And remember, boys are less well equipped than girls to exchange information between hemispheres. This includes being able to apply the nonverbal cues (which include, for example, the tone and volume of speech) detected by the right hemisphere to the more linear processing of language going on in the left hemisphere. A mother recently told me about an outing with her five-year-old twins, Cameron and Chloe. "We were at the park, and two kids, a brother and sister, walked up near them. The girl looked at them and said in a funny voice to her brother, 'Hmm, I just wonder who wants to play with us,' and they ran off to the slides. Chloe immediately got it and yelled, 'Hey, you silly guys, wait up for me!' Cameron loves the slides, but I had to tell him he could go over to play too."

Expressive language contributes to the development of social intelligence because being verbally expressive provides opportunity for social interaction, leading to the type of experiential opportunities critical to developing an awareness of how people relate. A boy who seldom speaks with peers is not learning from trial and error how his words affect others. In contrast, a boy who is involved in a lot of verbal give and take is more likely to learn how his words and behavior are perceived. Through practice and repetition, he gains a more sophisticated awareness of when his communication and behavior will be positively or negatively acknowledged. This type of social intelligence contributes to the development of both prosocial behavior and emotional literacy.

> ■ ■ ■
>
> You can reinforce and encourage a positive trajectory from social intelligence to positive social behavior by helping your son relate his communication style to specific consequences, good or bad. "It was smart of you to notice that Darien was upset about being chosen last, and I know she appreciated what you said to her about it. I wonder if next time you might say something to the other kids about wanting Darien on your team before sides get picked. That's part of being a team captain."

What about children who have expressive language skills but don't use their words kindly? Most of us can probably recall a school bully whose power may have been heightened by a certain degree of charisma and self-confidence. Boys like this can "read" others and can potentially use their verbal skills to manipulate or hurt other children. Bullies may possess a kind of social intelligence but lack the empathy to use their power in a constructive way. Their good perceptual or communication skills do not result in emotional literacy or ethically minded (prosocial) behavior. Bullies often emerge when there is an absence of clear moral leadership at home or if boys perceive that there are status advantages to asserting their dominance. As we discussed in the last chapter, early and intensive intervention will be required to help these boys. Overall, it may be easier to help a boy whose social and communicative difficulties are more brain related than characterological, because usually the environment can be shaped to meet the needs of the former.

The Emerald City: Emotional Intelligence

I first became aware of the extraordinary emotional impact of listening skills and phonological processing several years ago. At that time I was working with men, often referred to me for anger management, marital problems, or a related difficulty with getting along with others. In addition to the situational problems these men faced, most of them had substantial trouble with what we call emotional intelligence, a combination of both social intelligence and emotional literacy. They usually had difficulty detecting or understanding the emotions of others and lacked intuitive knowledge about how to use their own emotions constructively. One man was in disbelief that his wife had left him simply because he needed to punch holes in walls every now and then! It was painful to see the prevalence of unintentional social mistakes these men made and how hard it was for them to "unlearn" the behavioral reflexes that shaped their unsatisfactory relationships and social lives. One of the most frequent problems I observed was how loud they became when they wanted to make what they felt was an important point. Instead of drawing people closer to their thoughts, their loud volume pushed people away. For other men, learning not to "shut down" when they got angry was their biggest challenge. They wondered why others got frustrated with their silence, assuming that others knew what their silence meant. Unfortunately, most of these men were prone to repeating their mistakes, which, as I've described, often centered on their awkward or unaware communication style. Although most of them had never been formally identified as having a learning disability, one could make a strong argument that their difficulties reflected an inability to grasp the language of emotions. It was as though their brains had a "blind spot" for emotional learning.

In therapy, I noticed what I thought was a peculiar trait shared by many of these men—a tendency to mispronounce words. At first I believed it was just an interesting observation and didn't think much of it. As I became more aware of the behavior, I started making notes about what I heard. For example, I noted that while words might be mispronounced, they were used in the correct context. The speaker knew what the word meant. For example, the phrase "Let me tell you my perspective" would include the pronunciation of *perspective* as though it should sound like "pur-pos-pective." Usually, the words tended to be relatively common: *erroneous* ("air-ran-ee-us") *continuity* ("con-toot-y"), *inconsistent* ("in-con-sis-i-tant"), *interrogate* ("intro-grate"), and so forth. These were words that anyone watching the evening news or having normal conversations might be expected to know. Then, if I incorporated one of these words into a conversation with the correct pronunciation, I noticed my patients never gave me a double take or any other type of indication that they felt I was mispronouncing the word. Finally, when they had occasion to use the word again, they did not alter their own pronunciation. It seemed to be a peculiar form of "deafness," whereby they simply did not hear the pronunciation difference.

At the same time, I began informally investigating phonological processing and how poor awareness of word sounds might logically contribute to mispronunciation. Let's consider the critical link between auditory skills like phonological awareness and the capacity to develop social skills and emotional intelligence. The link makes sense, because if people do lack adequate auditory processing for the subtleties that shape word sounds, they are unlikely to appreciate the different kinds of inflections used in speech and the different ways words are used to convey meaning. It is as though an entire dimension of interpersonal communication is lost. As a result, language may be reduced to being more utilitarian or instrumental, lacking the emotional nuances that enable a full spectrum of thoughts and feelings. In essence, effective listening skills provide invaluable cues about the meaning of what is communicated. Processing speech and language without these skills is akin to reading sentences composed of nouns and verbs but lacking the descriptive benefit of adjectives.

In fact, someone may be so ineffective in hearing and remembering language that his own words have the opposite effect of what he intends. One of my adult clients frequently mangled common expressions. At one point, he related the details of a heated disagreement he had had with his boss, during which he exclaimed, "That bakes the cake!" When his boss responded with laughter, he was outraged that his indignation seemed to be met with derision. He had no idea that his words had undermined the seriousness of his argument.

It's almost impossible to overstate the importance of auditory processing skills in developing good expressive and receptive communication skills. We've witnessed the arrival and departure of a number of theories about the causes of syndromes such as dyslexia. However, our current understanding of phonological processing, as a formative component in the development of reading and good communication skills, will likely continue to command the attention of researchers in educational psychology.

Does Your Son Have a Nonverbal Learning Disability?

Although most learning disabilities involve some kind of reading impairment, nonverbal learning disabilities (NLDs) are an important consideration when it comes to appreciating the learning difficulties of many boys. NLDs frequently have an impact on social competence, particularly the ability to understand nonverbal communication. Based on my experience in working with school-age boys, I would suggest that NLDs are underdiagnosed and underappreciated for how they impair boys' social self-concept. The NLD syndrome, which is believed to affect primarily the brain's right hemisphere, typically includes impairment in one or more of the following four areas: motor skills/coordination, spatial perception and organization, social interaction, and poor sensory acuity in one or more of the five senses. As you can see, nonverbal learning challenges include a fairly diverse group of potential perceptual and behavioral deficits.

Because NLDs may not impact academic performance as dramatically as other learning disabilities, they may not generate the same degree of concern in school. Yet nonverbal learning disabilities tend to affect boys systemically, undermining social skills and self-esteem that help make learning possible. Making matters worse, such deficits may not be detected until boys are older, when symptoms are more pronounced.

Of particularly high relevance to boys of few words, NLDs often include problems with what is called *pragmatic communication*. Before we discuss this concern, a word of caution: "syndromes" and their associated symptoms exist on a continuum. You don't have to have been diagnosed with an NLD to be challenged by pragmatic communication skills. Many boys struggle with social learning skills, including those who are intelligent and academically successful. Ironically, boys with *exceptionally* high intelligence may be especially prone to social deficits, due to their typical preference for internalized (that is, self-reflective, analytical, abstract) thinking. Parents of a gifted child are right to monitor his social progress; his native intelligence can potentially impede his chances for "popularity" and social acceptance.

You can take heart, however, in knowing that intelligence can also be a great resource in learning how to crack the code of pragmatic communication.

> ■ ■ ■
> Coaching boys with nonverbal learning disabilities to social success means creating ample opportunity to rehearse practical communication skills.

Show your son how to make an introduction, for example, and then go over the steps in anticipation of meeting a new person. Encourage your son to use his new skills whenever an opportunity comes up.

Pragmatic Communication: Knowing the Rules of Engagement

Communication pragmatics involve knowing the rules and conventions that apply to different social situations. Communication occurs in contexts that change, and as the situations change, so does communication style. An overview of some of these rules and conventions, along with examples of how these skills might be impaired, is on the next page. Examples of pragmatic communication include learning how to take turns in a conversation (not interrupting or "talking over" someone else), appropriately modulating volume (boys should know they may be louder in the cafeteria than in the classroom), and knowing how to modify language depending on who the other person is (for example, a classmate versus the school principal). Others may perceive boys who don't understand the conventions of pragmatic communication as annoying, unintelligent, or aggressive.

FIGURE 2. Pragmatic (practical) communication skills.*

Skill	Possible problems
Physical	
Maintaining appropriate conversational distance	Other children may complain that "he's bothering me," or say "tell him to stop touching me" while playing together. Sometimes inserts himself physically into a group of children by pushing or nudging others out of the way in order to join the conversation.
Eye contact	Doesn't look others in the eye; hides behind hair/hat/sunglasses; stares to the point of discomfort.
Linking gestures with ideas and emotions	Body language doesn't match speech (thanks you for giving him a desired gift but slumps and stares off into space); waves too strongly or too unenthusiastically for the circumstances; forgets to reinforce emotion with body language.
Using facial expression effectively	Facial expressions don't convey interest in other people; expression is not congruent with topic or situation; doesn't nod to show he gets the point, looks furious at small disappointment; forgets to smile
Verbal	
Attending to time and place	Talks too fast; doesn't know when to interject a comment or let others speak, doesn't know how much information to share (goes on and on about a subject to someone's obvious irritation).
Turn taking	Consistently interrupts; doesn't perceive when it's someone else's turn to talk.
Voice modulation	Has trouble with prosody (pitch, tone, volume, inflection); speaks too softly or loudly without regard for physical proximity (you're across the room but he doesn't raise his voice to answer you).
Giving compliments	Doesn't know how to give a compliment relevant to a person and circumstances; sometimes unintentionally insults people ("You're a lot less fat than you were").
Greetings and good-byes	Doesn't know how to introduce himself to individuals or groups; can't initiate social contact (avoids parties and gatherings); doesn't know how to close a conversation (just walks off when he's done talking); doesn't shake hands/share hugs with close friends or family members; forgets to say "hello."
Thinking	
Detecting emotions in other people	Doesn't consider other people's emotional state before speaking (you're in the middle of an argument with someone and he asks you to make him a snack); doesn't realize when it's time to "back off"; doesn't read signs about how you feel (thinks you're mad when you're not).
Perceiving and expressing humor	Takes jokes, sarcasm or irony literally; laughs at inappropriate times; doesn't engage in word play or friendly teasing with peers.
Knowing how to make conversational transitions	Forgets to take his turn in conversations (calls you up on phone and then says nothing); discussions filled with uncomfortable "dead space"; doesn't pick up on "leads" to continue conversation (So, you like baseball? Who's your favorite team?).
Anticipating other people's reactions	Neglects to consider the impact of his words before speaking; can't easily imagine how his words or actions will be perceived by others (says he likes one present more than another at his birthday party without anticipating that someone's feelings will be hurt).

*All these skills should be considered in an age-appropriate context. Many of these skills are developed in adolescence. Compare your son's abilities relative to his peers'.

Pragmatics also involve the awareness and comprehension of nonverbal communication. The inability to "read" nonverbal behavior has been named *dyssemia* by psychologists Stephen Nowicki Jr. and Marshall Duke in their informative book *Helping the Child Who Doesn't Fit In.* This important nonverbal perceptual deficit is a significant liability in forming friendships and other relationships.

Anthony, a prominent real estate developer, told me about an incident with his eight-year-old son, Tony Jr., that occurred at his country club's family day. "Tony's got this thing where he gets needy or something and starts hugging people. It was cute when he was three, but it's time he grew out of it!" complained his

■ ■ ■
Most of us can respond to someone's nonverbal communication and respond accordingly. For example, if you're interviewing for a job and the interviewer frowns, folds her arms, and leans back, you may modify your statements or change course. If the interviewer leans forward, smiles, and nods, you may conclude that you're doing well and use that information to your benefit. A boy with an NLD may not notice that a peer is becoming impatient with his monologue on the mechanics of a snowblower. Boredom in facial expressions or the impatience in a rapidly tapping foot may go virtually undetected.

father. While the other boys played in the pool, Tony had circulated among the tables at a barbecue and kept climbing on people's laps and giving hugs. Anthony was embarrassed by his son's behavior and winced when Tony insisted on hugging an important business colleague. "She said, 'Oh, I like you too,' but she was obviously uncomfortable with it—she hardly knew him. When I led Tony away, his eyes teared up. I told him he shouldn't hug people he hardly knows, and he told me, 'But she said she liked me.' Tony just doesn't *get* it—he doesn't understand the difference between how you act with family and people who are practically strangers. I'm worried about what other people think of him!"

Anthony was right in observing that Tony didn't get it. He didn't perceive the situational code for appropriate social boundaries and took his father's colleague's words quite literally, totally failing to read her body language—a form of nonverbal communication. For boys with impaired pragmatics, a large social gathering can be very intimidating. Tony may have been seeking reassurance and connection but was unable to get it because he had trouble perceiving the social conventions at work and didn't understand that his actions were likely to be perceived unfavorably.

It's not hard to imagine that boys like Tony will often feel confused and anxious in groups, because so many situations will seem socially ambiguous to them. Most of us probably err on the side of being conservative when we're unsure of the social conventions in a new environment, restricting demonstrative communication until we understand what's normal for the group. But boys with pragmatic communication difficulties lack the fundamental interpersonal awareness that provides this type of "check and balance." *You can't find an answer if it doesn't occur to you to ask a question.*

Parents who don't witness the kind of behavior Tony engaged in may not realize right away that their son has a pragmatic communication problem. Eleven-year-old Michael had repeatedly complained to me about his difficulty making friends and how baffled he was that he was not more popular. During our meetings, no matter how much I tried to probe the issue, Michael could only respond with "I don't know, they just don't like me—there's no reason," and he always seemed very nice and well behaved. But when I went to his school to observe him in his normal daily surroundings, I was surprised to see Michael rushing down the hallways with his head down, shoulders drawn forward, and arms rigid. He looked unapproachable, even intimidating, and his peers literally and emotionally learned to stay away. He was so absorbed in his own thoughts, and anxious to get to the next class, that he didn't realize the nonverbal message he was sending.

For the next few weeks we practiced walking around the halls of my office building, smiling at people we passed and pausing to exchange greetings. (We also discussed context—Michael knew not to stop and chat with strangers in unfamiliar places.) This small skill had a clear, positive result for him in school. In essence, Michael had been introduced to an important part of the code for gaining social acceptance. As concerned parents, one of the things you can do is to stop, look, and listen and just observe your son with friends or at school. It can be very enlightening—we all tend to modify our behavior according to the circumstances, so your son may act differently outside his home environment. And you can help your son practice small skills just as Michael and I did.

Helping boys with nonverbal learning challenges is difficult but

can be successful. Social skills training for children usually emphasizes intensive instruction in social pragmatics. However, even with
repeated rehearsal, some boys have great difficulty integrating this
knowledge and making
it as automatic as would
be advantageous in most
social situations. It's not
that these boys can't make
progress, but we are asking
them to develop skills in
an area where they lack
natural ability. Patience
and persistence are the
keys here. Part of the chal-
lenge of teaching social skills to boys is overcoming their frequent resistance to taking direction from others. If we simply call attention to
a boy's social deficits, we risk heightening his self-consciousness and,
by extension, his defensiveness.

■ ■ ■

Will your son's school allow you to
observe him in school in a way that will
be acceptable to his teacher and not place
him in an embarrassing position?
Possibilities include volunteering in his
class, helping to monitor a gym or recess,
and attending a special program.

As hard as it might be for boys to accept feedback from adults, it
can be even harder for them to hear criticism from peers or siblings.
Oliver, a ten-year-old boy whose mother had recently married a man
with two children from a former marriage, was having difficulty with
his new stepsiblings, Meredith, nine, and Curran, twelve. Stepsibling
relationships are a common challenge for blended families, but when
we had our first family session the causes of Oliver's problems became clearer. For example, Oliver frequently complained that Curran

■ ■ ■

Diagnosing a Nonverbal Learning Disability

NLDs may come to light in several different ways, one of which is the
presence of dyssemia and related forms of social awkwardness. For other
boys, problems with spatial perception or math will be a prominent symptom.
The diagnosis of an NLD requires a thorough investigation of right-
hemisphere-driven skills. There could be a pervasive problem with such skills,
or the concern might be more focused. This type of learning disability requires
substantial expertise with NLD symptoms. Even today, some schools are
unclear that this is a legitimate type of learning disability that requires
accommodation and intervention.

was "bossy." When the family entered my office, Oliver immediately sat in my desk chair, while the rest of the family moved toward the sofa and chairs where we hold family sessions. Curran, concerned that Oliver was sitting at my desk, gave me a worried peek and said to him quietly, "Oliver, why don't you go sit there?", indicating one of the other chairs. Oliver stomped over to the chair, muttering, "You can't tell me what to do." Meredith, a bit nervous about the meeting and on her best behavior, promptly "shushed" Oliver. When he scowled, she touched his elbow and tried making a silly face. "She's picking on me!" he exclaimed. Oliver wasn't following their efforts to keep him "out of trouble." Instead, he misread their motivations and behavior. These types of interpretive errors are not uncommon among boys with social learning deficits and can be exacerbated in situations where boys feel vulnerable and tense. A good strategy in situations that heighten feelings of vulnerability is to make it a point to elicit a boy's opinion or insight, especially when you suspect he will be able to reply successfully. It's not unlike the way game show contestants are sometimes asked very simple questions at first, to help them get over the jitters and fear of failure. By doing this we limit the adverse impact of social learning deficits on self-esteem. When parents consistently employ strategies like this, the likelihood of being able to kindly communicate their most serious concerns is much greater.

Socially Indifferent

Some boys affected by a learning disability are not highly social, yet they aren't typically antisocial either. Instead, they are better described as *asocial*. They may be rather indifferent to social interaction as the result of either not perceiving the value of being social or simply having been exposed to so many situations in which they felt inept that they have given up on the possibility of social success! Martin spoke of his frustration with his sixteen-year-old son, Brian, whom he had lent money to buy his first car. The money was lent with the stipulation that Brian would get a summer job and begin paying back a portion of the loan. In one month, Brian had been fired from two jobs. He lost his first job at a hardware store because, in the words of his manager, "he hid from the customers" and was perceived as being curt by other employees. Brian was fired from the second job at a garden center because he was frequently late, which

184 ■ ESPECIALLY CHALLENGING BOYS

meant the girls he worked with had to take over his assigned task of hauling the heavy potted plants out to the front of the store at the start of the day. "The girls got irritated, and rightly so—he showed no consideration for them," complained Martin. "He's got no responsibility!"

Meeting with Brian, I realized it wasn't that he was trying to avoid work, but that he was truly confused about workplace expectations and consequences. "I'm a big screw-up," he said. The remark was enough to get my attention, but I found myself even more concerned by the matter-of-factness with which he made it. It felt as though he didn't care about his pattern of mistakes and had already resigned himself to the probability of future failures. What possible payoff does a boy get from "dropping out" of trying? Why doesn't he try harder? Isn't he concerned about what other people think? What *does* he care about?

When we ask questions like these, we're looking for psychological answers. Yet the genesis of the problem for boys with learning disabilities lies in the brain's idiosyncrasies and the behavior that results from those unique differences. Consequently, more often than not, the clearest path across the communication divide requires a long-term commitment to the development of self-management skills.

Wired for Distraction: ADHD

Affecting many of the boys described in this book is a syndrome so pervasive that its acronym—ADHD—has entered the lexicon of family life. ADHD's benchmark symptoms such as fidgeting, distraction, and impulsivity, are a major part of the behavioral equation for many young boys. They are also fairly familiar to the public, and they're likely to be the reasons parents have their sons evaluated for ADHD in the first place. Less frequently discussed is the impact of ADHD on social interaction and communication, yet I believe these difficulties are some of the most distressing effects of ADHD to boys themselves.

ADHD can make it more difficult for your son to make and keep friends, not just because his impulsivity can make it hard for him to adhere to social conventions like waiting his turn and being tactful, but because of a much more fundamental scattered communication style that ADHD can cause. If your son has ADHD or you suspect he might, you may already be aware of how disruptive many children with the syndrome can be at school. This too is a socially significant problem. The social consequences of ADHD across a variety of settings can be far-reaching, causing low self-esteem and ultimately despair, anger, or indifference.

When ADHD is a concern, you'll be able to complement the efforts of your son's teachers and health care practitioners by paying specific attention to his social and communication deficits, starting with a thorough understanding of how they operate. Understanding how ADHD creates these deficits may also help you decide to have your son evaluated for the disorder if you're not sure why your son is a boy of few words.

■ *Boys with ADHD can't explain their behavior—but it's usually not premeditated.* Talking to boys about the disruptive misbehavior of ADHD is typically an exercise in frustration. Our questions may be the obvious ones, "Why did this happen?" or "Why do you think you did that?" And the replies are nearly always the same: "I don't know, I just did it." Although I believe that boys can successfully take control of their behavior, at least more than they think they can, we should appreciate that there is not generally a premeditated thought process that leads to their misbehavior. The triggers for ADHD behavior may be environmental, but vulnerability to those triggers is rooted in neurodevelopment. Keeping this in mind may ease your frustration in trying to talk to an inattentive or hyperactive boy.

■ *Attention deficits have a considerable impact on expressive language development.* In boys, ADHD is typically associated with a high degree of impulsivity, which undermines thoughtful processing of speech and language. In the Mighty Good Kids™ groups that I run for boys with ADHD, I frequently witness this problem in the initial sessions. One boy will find the courage to make an important self-disclosure, but before he is even finished, another boy will react with a comment that is unrelated and often disrupts the potential for emotional connection. Working with these boys requires frequent prompting and redirection of their communication. As demanding as this can be, it's a good opportunity to apply the principle of behavioral bidirectionality—by asking these boys to slow down and consider what they want to say, parents and professionals are encouraging the interpersonal awareness so important to achieving social milestones like friendship.

■ *The hyperactivity of ADHD is antithetical to the focus required for good, reciprocal communication.* The helter-skelter processing of information that comes with ADHD leads to substantial social deficits. Boys with hyperactivity have difficulty incorporating social observations and what they hear in conversational speech into their own behavior. Parents of boys with ADHD have often seen the social consequences firsthand. Although many boys with ADHD have social inclinations, their ability to follow through appropriately on those interests and to structure relationships with peers constructively is often quite limited. Complicating this situation are the impulsivity and related behavioral attributes of these boys, which can cause them to be shunned by peers.

Boys are frequently both frustrated and perplexed by the dilemma. John, age ten, got very upset when I asked him about his relationships with friends at school. John said he liked other kids, and they liked him too, but they always ended up fighting. John's mother interjected that "the kids really do like him, but they also get frustrated by him." John had difficulty respecting interpersonal boundaries and was often over physical with other children at school. When John got very excited, as he was often inclined to do, he would encroach on his classmates personal space, talking over them and eventually causing them to retreat. It was difficult to convey this information to John, as his impulsivity made it obviously difficult for him to absorb and retain information on this level.

> ■ ■ ■
>
> Tapping in to your son's visual, auditory, and kinesthetic senses will enhance his ability to learn pragmatic social skills. Teachers who work with learning disabled children are usually very adept at communicating on multiple levels to maximize their learning potentials.

Executive Mismanagement

The difficulty of converting an intellectual concept into a behavioral change comes up over and over again with ADHD boys. While they may have the cognitive resources to fully understand a concept, the effects of hyperactivity and impulsivity make it difficult to absorb that information in a way that changes their behavior. This is the essence of what is called an *executive control* deficit. Executive control refers to abilities that originate in the brain's prefrontal cortex, which is a part of the brain's frontal lobe. This part of the brain is responsible for coordinating and facilitating the mechanics of attention and concentration. The relationship of executive control to the whole brain has often been described as being like that of a conductor of an orchestra getting all the musicians to play in concert. In addition to attention, some of the important executive functions enabled by the prefrontal cortex include the ability to shift focus from one thing to another (and back again when appropriate), planning and organization, short-term memory, emotional regulation, and the ability to self-monitor. Effective communication requires many of these skills. For example, to effectively lead a conversation you have to know where you're going—you have to plan and organize your thoughts and speech. In addition, the ability to self-monitor is critical to gauging how your communication is affecting someone else. An important part of development for all children is the process of becoming more reflective than reactive—this development is at the heart of self-awareness and, by extension, self-control. And this development is precisely what boys with ADHD find so difficult and why their communication is often unconsidered.

Part of the reason that boys with ADHD are impulsive is their inability to be aware of the consequences of their behavior; they don't necessarily relate an action in the present with an outcome in the future. Another particularly difficult challenge for boys with ADHD, highlighted in the research and writing of neuropsychologist Russell Barkley, is the management of time. Many dimensions of time management hinder these boys, including the challenge of doing age-appropriate tasks consistently without constant reminders. Twelve-year-old Tristan is an example. The next-door neighbors hired him to take care of their

> ■ ■ ■
>
> The brain's *executive control* functions include the ability to shift focus, plan, and organize, in addition to short-term memory, emotional regulation, and self-monitoring. A child with executive control problems often benefits when someone can act as a "surrogate," providing needed prompts and reminders. Your son will need you to remind him of the steps involved in greetings and good-byes, social conversation, and compliments: "Donovan, remember to look at Grammy when you say good-bye, and I know she'll appreciate it if you give her a hug too."

dog while on vacation. Tristan's mother was a bit concerned about the responsibility but was eager for opportunities that might help him mature. It was agreed that he would check on the dog before school, immediately after school, and once again in the evening. Tristan's mother came home from work one night to find him sobbing hysterically, saying that he'd killed the dog. She ran next door, to find the dog alive but semiconscious, and raced it to the vet. It turned out that although Tristan gave the dog its required medication each day, he did not give it consistently at the same time of day, as the dog's owners had emphasized. The dog eventually recovered, but the relationship with the neighbors did not. In hindsight, his mother said, "I don't know why I agreed to let him do this. He can't do his household chores unless I stand there and supervise him." Inadvertently, what had seemed like an opportunity to build Tristan's self-respect had backfired. Tristan would likely have done better if he were required to frequently verbalize his understanding of the instructions he had been given about taking care of the dog. Being asked to articulate those steps in a sequential manner would have helped Tristan transfer instructions from short-term memory to long-term memory—precisely what's required to remember to do something.

In One Ear, Out the Other

ADHD is also highly related to a lack of auditory processing skills. This may explain the strong relationship between ADHD and certain types of learning disability (researchers estimate that as many as 50–70 percent of children with ADHD also have a learning disability, although this is a difficult statistic to pin down because of divergent criteria for determining learning disabilities), most notably those requiring phonological processing. Sometimes auditory processing is affected by a poor short-term memory, which means that as boys learn new information they don't retain it long enough for it to be fully encoded and available for retrieval hours, days, or weeks later. "In one ear, out the other" is how it's manifested: Rashid gets sent to the store one block away and forgets what he's supposed to bring home; Alan can't remember where he put his homework; Dante doesn't recall the time of his curfew. This is one reason so many boys can be frustrating to adults. Boys will be taught something, appear to understand the instructions clearly, and then the next day be unable to remember what steps or sequence of actions they should follow to complete the necessary task. Adults, perceiving that the boys are fully capable of performing the task, sometimes get angry with these boys, mistakenly believing their problem lies in attitude. To be sure, it can be difficult to figure out if someone "forgets on purpose" or if a lack of motivation is contributing to the problem. However, the ability to sequentially remember instructions is a core component of executive control.

The Social Challenges of ADHD

In more recent years, research has begun to focus on how ADHD affects communication skills. In a 2002 *Journal of Child Psychology and Psychiatry* study, psychologists Cheryl Clark, Margot Prior, and Glynda Kinsella found that adolescents with executive control problems (ADHD) had greater problems with adaptive communication (pragmatics) than peers who had been diagnosed as having serious behavioral problems. The researchers also found that the social competence of teenagers with ADHD and conduct disorder was about the same, with both groups demonstrating marked deficiencies. These findings reflect that ADHD is a source of both communication and social problems.

Tara, a new teacher, was telling me about a boy in her class. "Neil is just one of those kids who gets my back up, and I feel really bad about it. I know he has problems, but when he walks in the door, I tense up. He's always in the middle of a problem, causes so many interruptions, he needs so much. He was home sick for a week, and it was like a vacation for the whole class—isn't that awful? I love kids. I don't want to feel this way about him."

While boys with ADHD may draw negative attention primarily because of undercontrolled behavior, these boys are clearly more than "problems to be managed." We need to take seriously how hyperactivity shapes the way boys think and feel about themselves and others. Hyperactivity can make it a challenge to slow down long enough to recognize that other people matter and notice that they require personal attention. TJ, a rambunctious nine-year-old, upset his parents when he snatched his birthday present from his aunt's hand, tore it open, and immediately ran out to the yard to play with his gift. "It happened in one minute flat—zoom! He was gone!" exclaimed his mother.

For yet other boys, whose ADHD is primarily a problem with

distractedness, the key challenge is helping them give adequate attention to their social environment. To these boys, people may matter much less than personal interests or even their moment-to-moment fascination with passing thoughts or observations. Consider Tyrus, who upset his parents by hardly acknowledging their houseguests while he played his GameBoy nonstop. "When he brought it to dinner, that was the last straw. I locked it up," said his dad. Unfortunately, it's not possible or practical to "lock up" all the potential sources of distraction that boys like Tyrus can find. It's not that limiting a boy's involvement with distracting pursuits is necessarily wrong, but the development of sufficient social skills requires more than parentally imposed rules. It also requires social interest. None of us develops an interest because we're required to by some higher authority. Social interests grow from life experience and our natural curiosity about other people. The neuropsychology of ADHD seems to obstruct the kind of awareness that would promote healthy social interest. Not surprisingly, a lack of curiosity about other people limits the motivation to communicate. For parents, it helps to be aware of the social deficits that often accompany ADHD when considering diagnosis and treatment options.

> ■ ■ ■
> Awareness of others fosters healthy social interest and motivates communication. Sometimes hyperactivity can make it a challenge to slow down long enough to recognize that other people matter and notice that they require personal attention.

It May Take a Team

Significant questions remain about how parents and professionals can and should help children with ADHD. My concern here is the impact the syndrome is having on the social development of so many boys and, ultimately, the impact it will have on their lives as men. Because of that impact, I hope what you've read so far has convinced you not to ignore ADHD in the hope that your son will outgrow it— or to address only the academic problems that ADHD brings.

For some boys affected by ADHD, medication has made a critical difference in the development of self-regulation, school achievement, and the self-esteem that results from prosocial behavior. Behavior management and social skills training have helped boys control their

Learning and Attention Problems ■ 191

behavior and get along at school and elsewhere. But like many psychologists I've learned that it may take a team to help a boy with ADHD avoid the potentially damaging frustration and devastating self-esteem problems that the syndrome can cause.

Colin had had "possible ADHD" noted on his progress reports since sixth grade, but it wasn't until he reached his freshman year in high school that his grades began to fall sharply. Under pressure from his school, Colin's father brought him in for an evaluation. He had resisted in the past because he thought his son would outgrow the problem, and until Colin's grades fell drastically, he didn't believe there was much of a problem to begin with. I asked him to consider the specific social concerns raised by Colin's teacher: his tendency to "overpower" other students, speaking impulsively in class, and giving the impression that he was rarely interested in what anyone else was saying. One of the lowest moments of the evaluation, that Colin's father ultimately agreed to, occurred when I escorted Colin back to my waiting room following what he found to be a series of particularly exasperating tests. "Dad, I can't do it. You don't understand. I'm failing. I have no friends. I'm like a freak," he said.

"Are you trying?" replied his father. "I sincerely don't understand what your problem is."

"Yes, I'm trying! What do you want from me? Just forget it," Colin mumbled. Colin's self-esteem had tanked, to the point of wanting to give up and withdraw.

After Colin was tested, his father and I met to review the results. We talked about Colin's difficulty in slowing down his thoughts and communication. Our discussion focused on the social consequences of Colin's condition, which were heightened by statements Colin had made at various points during evaluation—"Kids think I'm mean, but I'm not," "I'm sick of making mistakes," and "Can you make me grow out of this?" Once Colin's father realized how ADHD was affecting his son emotionally, he was very committed to helping him. He agreed to speak with a physician about the pros and cons of medication, and we discussed ways that he could provide effective modeling and encouragement for Colin.

Complicating the situation was the fact that Colin's father was a single dad who worked long hours. Effective behavioral interventions require an extraordinary level of commitment and consistency on the part of family. Fortunately, we were able to enlist the participation of two teachers, who began monitoring Colin for both behavioral concerns like inattention and impulsivity and social goals including elements of pragmatic communication.

If your son has ADHD, please keep in mind the importance of getting help from others—at school, in the medical community, and from counselors or therapists who know what boys with ADHD are up against. You will likely ask yourself in frustration how you're supposed to build in structure, help your son follow a "behavior management chart," and mediate his social interactions when he is bouncing off the walls and you can't be there 24-7. But remember above all that communication is a learned behavior and that his potential for success will depend on having good teachers, parents, and professionals alike.

We Can Have an Impact

The boys described in Part II might be thought of as archetypal examples of boys of few words. They are the boys most vulnerable to short- and long-term life consequences, and they require all the love, intelligence, and effort we can muster to help them find the path of social success. If we don't attend to them as children, we'll be casting them adrift into a world that will likely respond to them with exasperation or hostility. The work we do can profoundly impact the quality of their lives and the lives of those around them, preventing social and communication deficits in boys of few words from escalating into long-term life limitations.

■ ■ ■

In Part III we will begin by examining core attributes of family life that can make a considerable difference to your son's healthy social development. I will describe a wide range of specific strategies designed to both prevent the emergence of problems and help boys develop the communication skills that increase their chances for social success. As we will see, there are many practical things that caregivers can do on a daily basis to plant the seeds of social awareness and to shape the language skills that lead to social acceptance. Part III will also discuss how to work constructively with your son's school and teachers to bring out the best in him at school—a child's most important social learning environment. Finally, we will review some suggestions about when you might need to seek a professional evaluation, and some specifics about what is involved in that process. We have already discussed much about the psychology and behavior of boys. The final leg of our journey will further help you translate that understanding into practical solutions that can make lasting differences in your son's life. There are many new ideas ahead, and I hope you will return to them often as your son grows into the fine young man he can be.

Part III

How to Make
Lasting Differences

...

EIGHT

Ten Commitments to Boys' Communication

■ ■ ■

I don't have to tell you that the strength and creativity of families is at the very heart of raising our sons well. I use the word *heart* quite intentionally, because a passion for parenting is an indispensable complement to informed, smart family leadership. You've already demonstrated your passion to see your son reach his potential as a social being by picking up this book. Although families are dynamic systems that differ in many ways, there are core commitments that define effective families. Your family will not necessarily adopt these commitments in the same way as other families might. Owing to circumstance and the individuality of family members, particularly parents, families inevitably discover the beat that synchronizes best with the dance of their members. Still, if you're to transform the course of your son's boyhood and ensure that he becomes a socially and emotionally healthy man, we need to look at how these individual commitments can help him build the expressive and social skills that will make him a happy and successful adult.

1. Making Time

Life changes when you have children, and so does your sense of time. In our multitasking, hectic, on-the-go world, making time is a tall order. But without time all the rest of our intentions will come to little. It's through making time that we demonstrate other people's importance in our lives. By giving of our time, we say to our sons, "You are important to me—you are my priority." Sometimes we make the mistake of trying to fill our children up with gifts, privileges, or even special experiences, but none of those things replaces the need for our time.

Making time also means more than simply doing something with your son. It means attending to him, noticing what he thinks and says, and responding to him in a way that makes him feel understood and important; these are skills he can "internalize" and use with others.

It can be relatively simple. Jenna, who shops at an upscale supermarket that provides a child care center for kids over age three, said, "I admit that when Nick was a baby, I looked forward to the time that I could drop him off while I shopped. But as he got older, I kept him entertained by talking about what we were buying, letting him help me pick out the vegetables, and letting him find items we needed. By the time he was old enough to go to the child care center, I realized that shopping is a fun thing that we both look forward to. We talk the whole time, and he's very proud of knowing how to pick out good produce and put it gently in the bags. He's a true companion!"

Jenna found a creative way to turn a chore into a pleasant ritual she could share with her son. Nick benefited in many ways, too. Along with using their shopping expeditions to teach basics such as colors and numbers ("Can you pick out three green apples?"), Jenna taught Nick that people like different foods (developing his appreciation that others may have a different like/perspective) and that he could take pride in finding items others would enjoy (consideration). As a "regular," he was befriended by the employees at the counters and checkouts, where they made a fuss over him, giving him a chance to develop his conversational skills. "Believe me, being known at the bakery counter as 'cookie man' is very cool for a three-year-old," said Jenna.

One of the keys to making time for children lies in the "downsizing" of life. When we reduce complexity and obligations, we feel less stressed in giving children the time they require. Establishing a family philosophy in which time spent with children is a priority, rather than an option or a plan for the future, is central to our success as parents. Since you've taken the time to read this book, I may well be "preaching to the choir." However, for a significant number of us, work is a major competitor for our time and attention. While most of us need to work to support our families, our perception of how much income we need, how important we are to our workplace, and how much time we should work outside the home is influenced by other factors. Sometimes those perceptions were formed before we became parents. It's usually surprising to new parents to discover both how very time-consuming, and rewarding, raising children is. Even if you stay at home with your child, things that were once accomplished in short order can take hours. Many of us have a script in mind for how we should live and what our work should be. Yet that script may have been written in our childhood or formed haphazardly from our observations of family and colleagues. Once we become parents, it may be time to thoughtfully reconsider that script.

It's particularly easy for men to be consumed by work, receiving a disproportionate amount of gratification and acknowledgment for activities unrelated to family life. As good as that acknowledgment feels, it sometimes has the unfortunate effect of leading us to increasingly emphasize the role of work in our lives. Maybe it's time that we learned to glean an equivalent level of satisfaction from the work of raising our children. What greater legacy can we hope to contribute to? Why is it that we don't always see how much our sons need us or how important we are to their social development? Making time for Little League games, scouting, and fishing is wonderful, but we also need to make time for imaginative floor play, parent–teacher meetings, helping with homework, teaching about dating and sex, and helping our sons discover who they are.

I often find myself saying to clients, "Life is not a dress rehearsal." If you reflect on how this statement relates to your current life, you may, like most of us, recognize that there are elements of the way you go about allocating time that don't reflect your true core values. In America, our focus on "time management" suggests an underlying belief that we need to be more efficient. This is a mistaken interpretation of our social situation. At some point, the pursuit of efficiency is a fool's errand because there is simply no more time to be had. The only way to meaningfully expand family time is to redefine priorities.

Think Like a Villager

You can also reframe what your family life feels like. To go back to Jenna and Nick, who shopped together, think about what you do in the presence of your children—everyday activities like cooking, cleaning, catching up on business, maintaining your car and yard, running errands, talking to friends. When we're pressed for time, it's easy to feel as though our kids are an impediment to efficiently working down our list of to-dos. Often, we're hurrying to get these things done so we can go play with our kids! Yet the division between the adult realm of responsibilities and that of children is sometimes artificial.

Imagine how families coped with everyday demands a few centuries ago. I'm not suggesting you put your son to work in the fields or send him out as an apprentice. Yet as we still see in some places in the world, where even young children are given responsibilities, boys are naturally integrated into the social fabric of their community. If you begin to think of your son less as a "responsibility" and more as a developing, resourceful member of your "clan," it's easier to imagine a role for him where social communication evolves organically.

Boys, who are very interested in how things work, often enjoy the chance to be a part of what you're doing. Whether it's washing the dog, shopping for your friend's birthday gift, or deciding how to budget for next year's vacation, if you include your son in the action and discussion, you build his sense of affiliation and help focus his attention toward the communal goals and interests of your family.

Of course, all this will take discussion and narrative from you. Suppose, for instance, that your mother is moving from her house into a seniors' apartment complex. You have to help her pack, put her home on the market, hire the movers, and offer her some reassurance throughout the process. Most of us have had to coordinate something complicated like this on top of our everyday experiences, and it's the kind of thing that eats up "child time." Yet if you include your son in the project, assuming he's old enough to help (let him set up the boxes, fold and pack, research realtors on the Internet, plot about tactful ways to introduce his grandmother to her new neighbors), you'll find plenty of opportunities to develop his social communication skills within the task-oriented realm so attractive to boys. And once you've included him in the project, you'll be able to introduce discussion that isn't so task oriented, but more focused on emotions: how you feel about your mother getting older, the memories you shared in the old house, your hopes and concerns about her new housing arrangement, tactful ways to ask her to throw out the junk in her garage, or even your own parent–child relationship.

Again, much of the success in reframing the activities of everyday life into an opportunity to connect with your son depends on your ability to narrate the experience for him. Sometimes when we're tired or busy, we don't want to take the time to explain what's on our mind or what we're doing. But you shouldn't underestimate a boy's interest in knowing how things work, especially adult concerns. "I'm clearing out the basement because I want to put in a woodworking shop" or "I'm cleaning the house like mad because my sister always teased me about being a slob when we were kids, and I don't want her to razz me when she gets here" can be a springboard for discussion and modeling. The great thing is that by incorporating these teachings into your everyday life, and including your son in activities that you would have been doing anyhow, you're not "losing" time. Why rush to get the car washed so you can drive your son to the water park? Invite your son to join you with a bucket of suds and admire how well he polishes. Have a water war. Tell him how you felt when you got your first car. The changes you're seeking may not happen overnight, but you'll open the door for them to happen.

No matter how your family handles the time issue, remember it's the one issue that you can't wait to resolve.

2. Empathy

Throughout this book I've emphasized the importance of nurturing the empathy of boys. Empathetic parenting means seeing each child as the unique individual he is. When you recognize the individuality of your son, you provide an acknowledgment he hungers for. You also stand in the best possible position to respond to his emotional needs. One demonstration of empathy is to respect that the way your son expresses himself tells you something important about who he is. We've explored how silence or awkwardness can be just as evocative as more extroverted communication styles. This is not to say that we should let the communication problems of our sons stand unchallenged, but empathy allows us to appreciate their differences from us and to hear, deeply, where they are coming from.

Empathy should also undergird parenting decisions. As a parent, you can model empathy by emphasizing the value of family members understanding one another. When your son senses that your intentions are authentic, and are thoughtfully motivated for the benefit of family relationships, his need to be resistant or defensive is diminished. When you articulate the value of empathy within the family, try to do so in a way that will be meaningful to your son. Boys tend to be unimpressed by vague abstractions such as "Be nice" or "It's the right thing to do."

Monica and Jay brought their sons, Cody, age nine, and Blain, age eleven, to see me. Their sibling rivalry had reached such a high pitch that the family was in turmoil. "They're impossible. They fight all the time. We tell them to cut it out, we treat them absolutely the same, but the complaints are constant!" said Monica. I was immediately interested when Monica said "we treat them the same" and asked why. "Well, we want to be fair," replied Jay. Our resulting conversation explored the merits of treating the boys differently—at least in some respects. If empathy means recognizing and reflecting another's individuality, then well-meaning attempts at "fairness," through equal treatment, may distract parents from important signals boys send about their needs. At any given time, these needs are unique. Blain was less articulate than his younger brother, so the family "agenda" was usually most influenced by Cody's requests. To put it simply, it didn't matter to Blain if they both got the same skateboard when he didn't particularly want one in the first place. The intense competition between the boys was spurred by their desire to be seen and treated as individuals, rather than as interchangeable "units." I asked Monica what would happen if she did something special just with Blain. "I guess I'd feel guilty," she said with a smile.

"How would you feel if your mom or dad did something just with Blain?" I asked Cody. He thought about it. "I guess it'd be okay, if he was having a bad day or something," he replied. Cody understood that there would also be times when he would receive individual attention, although perhaps in a different way. We do our sons a great favor when we teach them about the complexity of concepts like fairness early in life.

Another aspect of empathy involves not allowing our interaction with children to be shaped by frustration or projection. Emily was telling me about her ex-husband's troubled relationship with their son, Randy. "Rob is in sales. He's tall, good-looking, articulate. He never said it, but the truth is that he's really disappointed not just in Randy's behavior, but in who Randy *is*. Randy isn't going to be the cool kid he takes to the club with him. He's not going to run for class president. He's short, he's shy, he has very different interests. Rob doesn't realize how vulnerable Randy is. When Rob talks about the things he *wishes* Randy was interested in, it makes Randy feel insignificant." It is nearly impossible to discover an empathetic approach to parenting if we are so intent on projecting our own values and needs that we lose sight of who our children are and consequently lose all capacity to help them become the best that they can be. Being a parent is by definition being a leader. To fulfill that role and provide guidance, we have to be able to transcend differences. When we try to provide a one-size-fits-all type of guidance we are misled and will, by extension, mislead our sons.

Being an empathetic parent also requires a significant amount of energy. In comparison with sympathy, empathy is far more active, requiring that we work hard at perceiving our sons' true selves. Although you may be reading this book believing that boys should be parented with specific social expectations, I hope you'll interpret the guidance in this book more as principles than as a set of rules. In accordance with your own son's or family's needs, you're likely to choose interventions or act on recommendations that are relevant to those needs. What is essential, however, is that you think carefully about what needs your son does have and apply yourself to meeting them in a way that respects his uniqueness. If you do that, you're acting empathetically.

3. Willingness to Take Action

It may seem obvious, but one of the key commitments that parents make is to be willing to do what is necessary to raise their sons well. This means acting on good intentions in a way that propels the healthy development of children and families. In most cases, *anticipatory action* is more useful than *reaction*. Our willingness to take action should begin when our sons are still young enough for us to have an impact on their social and emotional development. It may also require that we apply ourselves to working out parenting differences. When parents disagree about important concerns, family solidarity—an important foundation of our children's emotional security—is undermined. You may have resolved some of these concerns before your child was born, but by necessity new situations emerge that require parents to be co-problem-solvers.

Timing is an important consideration. Although you may know when to act, at least most of the time, at other times the answer to the question of "when" will be less obvious. If your son isn't talking to peers in preschool, you may decide to wait a while until he becomes more comfortable playing with others. If he's still not participating in kindergarten, you may need to consider intervention. If your fifth-grade son has an argument with a classmate, you may decide to let him try to handle it himself. If the conflict involves name calling or shoving, you may need to intervene. Certainly, the advice of a teacher or other parents can be helpful in unclear situations, especially if your child is unable, or reluctant, to explain the nature of his difficulties fully. However, because you know your son best, you are probably the best judge of when to step in. A good rule of thumb is to get involved when your son is unable to resolve the problem by himself and the situation is hurting him. Your intervention could be as mild as offering advice or as assertive as moving him to a new school; the art of parenting is knowing when and how to initiate action and, conversely, when to cease operations.

Negative behaviors that occur only intermittently can be the most confounding, because it's hard to tell if something is an anomaly (all kids do strange things at some times) or the start of a trend.

Sometimes the hardest part of taking action is having to accept that a particular intervention is required. Because parents tend to idealize their children, it may be hard for us to see and believe that they need help. When this is the case, a delay could be costly to a child's development. For example, many children are brought to therapy months or even years after the preferable time. Yet child development is so dynamic that it's possible to miss a window of opportunity. Ed, who was diagnosed with dyslexia as an adult, described it this way: "My mom was very soft-hearted. I didn't do good in school, and so she'd tell everyone, 'Stop picking on Ed, he's smart enough, he's good at other things.' I just thought I was stupid. Come to find out, there was a reason I couldn't read. She meant well, but my life would have been a lot different if I had found out sooner."

Part of being willing to take action is not being paralyzed by a fear of stigmatization. One of the positive changes of the last quarter century is how much less stigmatized families feel in accessing mental health care. Take the decisive steps required to address your son's needs, and avoid the trap of thinking that "he'll grow out of it." It may be years before your son realizes what you've done for him, but when he does, he will have a valuable insight for knowing how to parent his own children.

If you have a nagging feeling that your son's communication problems need attention but you don't know what to do, the next chapters may be of assistance, as we'll talk about the role of schools and when to seek professional help.

4. Staying Positive

A positive outlook is something our sons learn from and benefit from simultaneously. How do you "get positive"? With respect to supporting the communication development of our sons, getting positive means remaining optimistic in the face of difficulties or resistance to change. Although every child cannot accomplish all things, I've never met a child incapable of improvement. Being positive doesn't mean compelling someone to achieve amazing results through the sheer force of your will. Yet being positive does allow you to apply your understanding of your child and frame his potentials in a manner that points him toward success. Werner, a real estate executive, was working with his son, Leif, on being more sociable and mature at home. "He's seventeen and champing at the bit to get out of the house. He's tired of school. Every time he complained about it, I got so worried he'd let his grades slip that I would start lecturing him about the importance of continuing his education. He started shutting down. I changed my approach a little, and when he complained, I let him know that I felt the same way when I was in school. I told him about all the fun I had when I finally graduated and went off to college. Our conversations have turned around—now we talk about his 're-lease' and make plans for what he'll do in college. When I started treating him more like an adult, his behavior with me became more mature."

Staying positive also means you maintain a problem-solving perspective of whatever challenges your son faces. It's easy to get discouraged after repeated failures, and easy to give up if you feel as though success has come too slowly. Remember, however, that our children watch our reactions to their efforts very carefully. A boy who strikes out for the third time in a game is quick to glance at his parents in the stands and note if they look disappointed. In the same sense, it's important to stay positive about our sons' efforts in school, even if we feel such efforts haven't been as complete as they ought to be. I don't mean you need to overpraise a lackluster effort, but it's essential to notice and remark on improvements, even when small. Staying positive is a way of demonstrating faith and belief in our children. It may sound like something endemic to parenting, yet it's a principle that's easy to forget in the midst of stress and busy lives.

Cultivating a positive family atmosphere, of course, requires your child's other parent, if he has one, to be very positive as well. Cooperation between parents fuels your collective emotional energy, making you much stronger than either of you could be individually. We have already discussed how mood follows behavior. Positive words and actions have an effect on the whole family. When you take the time to say, "I like how you . . ."; "We noticed that you . . ."; "You're getting better at . . .", you're helping your son tune in to specific behaviors that you as a parent want to see, and you're also sensitizing yourself to his successes—and that's encouraging for you, too.

Being positive is not about putting on a superficial happy face. This is not a "fake it till you make it" philosophy. Our positive attitude must stem from connecting with the hope and the promise of our sons' lives. Is there any more basic emotional necessity that we owe our children? I can think of no greater threat to a family's well-being than emotional despair, because it leads to parenting inertia. Despair and depression are profound states of self-absorption, and families that find themselves in that emotional predicament are poorly positioned to provide leadership, solve problems, and plan for the future in the ways that families require.

If you notice your son struggling with his own belief in himself, or weighed down by emotional frustrations, check in with him. Children need to hear you say the words of encouragement and belief that seem obvious to you. Sometimes your child picks up doubts and worries from watching or listening to you; on occasion, he may misinterpret your words or actions and think something very bad has happened or that you're angry or upset with him. Maintaining a positive perspective begins with an individual commitment not to let your own emotional ups and downs become a defining element in the way you interact with your children. Parents should not feel required to hide their feelings, but our children should not be used as a sounding board for frustrations and problems that have little to do with them. Your ability to make positive acknowledgment a part of daily family life will provide the encouragement your son needs to eventually succeed on his own.

5. Being Informed

Although ultimately we all accept the responsibility for making decisions in our children's best interest, effective parents consider different ideas and perspectives and can learn and accomplish much by embracing the plurality of perspectives available. This includes information from both formal and informal sources. Formal sources could include reading current books, searching websites, or consulting a doctor. Equally important, however, is how we gain insight through more casual information networks. This might involve talking with friends, spending extra time at your son's school conferring with his coach, using your social network to share ideas and questions with others who may have valuable insight. Your relationship with your son's babysitter or his friend's parent may be an important complement to what you learn from professional sources. (Chances are you're the type of person who doesn't hesitate to access this information if you've gotten this far in this book.)

There is an art to sorting through the vast quantity of information available to parents. One valuable strategy is to identify a few trusted resources that you can return to repeatedly. This could be a newsletter about nonverbal learning disabilities or maybe a particular website that you find exceptionally helpful. I've also found that a very good principle is to seek a consensus of opinions. When you hear facts or ideas come up repeatedly, in different sources, you can probably trust there is some value in what you're reading. For example, you might read in several sources (books, websites, and a newsletter) that children with ADHD often have difficulty with expressive language and social skills. When you hear something like this often enough, it suggests that you're discovering an important fact that needs to be considered in more depth.

Finally, it's also necessary to allow your parenting to be shaped by new ideas. Sometimes important insights are counterintuitive, such as discovering that boys may compensate for social anxiety with loud or overbearing speech or that the taunting remarks of antisocial boys can make them more popular among peers. And sometimes we don't know what we think we know. Consider how many children with compromised reading skills were labeled as unintelligent before dyslexia became known and accepted. I believe similar disparities may currently exist regarding our understanding of social learning disabilities.

Another aspect of being informed is being assertive enough to get the information you need. *When you're meeting with professionals where complex ideas are being discussed, you must absolutely insist on a comprehensible explanation.* If you need more time for discussion, schedule a second appointment with your son's teacher, therapist, or doctor. Every profession—education, medicine, psychology—has its own terms and ideologies. You can weigh the merit of the advice you receive only if you're clear about what's being said. While evaluating a ten-year-old boy for learning disabilities, I asked his mother and her partner if his teachers ever mentioned any problems with auditory processing. The mother replied, "There were some notes on his report card to that effect, but we weren't really sure what they meant. Because we only have a lukewarm relation with his teacher, I didn't feel comfortable just picking up the phone and calling him to ask for clarification. I guess if they noticed something serious, the school would send a letter home."

The truth is, while most schools are very responsible about communicating with parents, it's not safe to assume that you're always on the same page or that you'll be informed of every problem your child has. Sometimes teachers second-guess their own perceptions as well. For example, a teacher might hesitate to mention that your son has difficulty making friends if you don't mention that you're having a similar problem in your neighborhood.

When I was a student learning how to administer psychological tests, we were asked to prepare a report based on our test administrations. I remember a long exchange between the professor and a fellow student. The professor kept asking, "What result did you get? What conclusion did you come to?" At each question, my classmate continued to list more statistical data. Finally, the professor snapped, "I can read the numbers! But what do the numbers *mean*?" A good professional will not only provide you with information, but will also provide recommendations and help you make an informed decision about how to help your child. A diagnosis (whether it's "Jeff is poor at calculations" or "Darrell has ADHD") is only a starting point.

Being informed is about more than collecting data. It's about pulling together the information you get from multiple sources to create a reliable portrait of your son. It's about knowing what resources are available to help you, and it's about keeping abreast of changes in your son's situation. As your son's parent, you're the CEO of decision making in his life. This is a role too important to delegate, and too important to manage based on guesswork or misinformation.

Let's get started. A list of resources you may find helpful is included at the back of this book.

6. Teaching

A large part of our role as parents is to provide for our sons' basic needs, from food and clothing to emotional necessities such as safety and love. Yet another important role is that of teacher. As teachers we impart not only "what" but also "why." We build our sons' social and self-awareness when we explain not only what we want them to do but why. It's surprising how often this very important and strategic parenting intervention gets neglected in the hustle and bustle of everyday life.

It's particularly easy to forget to explain social rules that may seem obvious to us. While adults might automatically link cause and effect for physical actions ("Get down—you could fall and get hurt!"), we might not say, "When you talk louder than everyone else, people can get irritated with you because they don't get a chance to be heard" or "When you interrupt John when he's talking, he thinks you don't care about what he's saying. He might get mad and decide not to listen to you."

This is not to say that we have to explain our every move or be misled into believing that our children should be equal to us in making important decisions. To do so would be impractical and potentially undermine our status as authority figures. But judiciously providing explanations shows respect for your child, because it gives him the information that will eventually enable him to make good judgments by himself. For example, if your boss pulls you off a project before it's complete and has you start another, you might think she's incompetent and feel irritated. If she levels with you about the departmental budget crisis, you might realize that the company has to cut its losses on the first project and agree that it's more strategic to work on the other task. Further, her explanation subtly indicates a degree of respect for your need to understand her decision. You may even have your own suggestions about improving matters. By the same token, we can expect a higher degree of insight and consideration from our children if we give them the tools to participate in family decision making.

It's particularly important to recognize the need of young children to understand why they are being asked to do something in a particular way. Matt and Paula were having a hard time getting their three sons, ages four, six, and seven, to pitch in around the house. "We had a rule that everyone should put his dirty clothes in the basket. Nobody was doing it," said Matt. "So we called a family meeting, and I said, 'We need your help. Mom helps the family by doing the laundry. It's a big job for one person. If we all share the work by putting our dirty clothes in the basket, she won't have to go into everyone's room to get them. That will make her happy, because she'll know we care about her.' Our youngest has really taken the job seriously, and he gets on his brothers if they forget. It was simple and it worked." When you provide answers about "why," you make your child a partner by helping him understand the principle that underlies whatever change you're trying to bring about.

Effective teachers choose their words in a way that builds collaboration. At a department store display of a Christmas tree full of ornaments, I saw the following interventions. One harassed mother said, "Keep your hands off those—you're gonna break something!" A few minutes later another parent said to her son, "These belong to the store until we buy one. Can you point to the ones you like?" The first boy could not be controlled and had to be carried, protesting, away from the display. The second child took the instruction in stride and enjoyed being asked his opinion. I suspected the second child was the beneficiary of frequent interaction with parents that reflected their respect for him. For practical reasons, teachers do best when they encourage the scaffolding of skills. If you want your child to learn how to make an introduction, then you need to start by teaching him to express a simple "hello" statement. This small skill can later be elaborated into a more complete introduction, including a question such as "How are you?" or "What do you want to do today?"

In the same sense, when we expect our teenage sons to act with conscience toward their community, we have the best chance if we teach the principles underlying such social commitment early in their lives. Scaffolding also requires that we reinforce positive changes, helping our sons feel pride in what they've already accomplished. In addition, by thinking out loud, we provide children with a window to our own thoughts and the kind of logic we use in solving problems or developing a new skill. Consequently, teaching is an excellent way to build insight in our sons. Teaching is about more than simply relating a set of skills; it's also about showing children *how to think*. Suppose your son tells you he's been offered a summer job by a cantankerous neighbor, and wanting time to think about it, he tells the neighbor he has to check with you first. You might reply, "I know that most people wouldn't mind waiting for an answer, but you noticed that Mr. Grimley sometimes takes offense easily, and you were smart to put it that way. If you decide to take the job, I don't think you'll have much trouble working for him, since you understand him so well." When we teach our children how to think in ways that build their self-confidence, we empower them to meet the challenges of adolescence and adulthood.

When parents are good teachers, they learn how to integrate principles and ideas into conversations with their children in a natural way. This requires learning to switch channels and pay close attention to the way boys are hearing you. We can look for cues in how they are hearing us in their facial expressions, eye contact, and all other visible indications of their comprehension. Instruction is also effective when presented in the form of a story.

Perhaps most important, the most effective and interesting teachers are eager students. If you've ever taught something to someone else, you know what I mean. When we teach other people, we tend to learn what we're teaching exceptionally well because we're required to think through an idea carefully enough to be able to explain it. That's one of the reasons why, when I'm trying to teach a child better self-control in school, I often suggest that he be made a mentor to another child with similar problems—to fulfill that role, he will by necessity have to explain the steps involved in achieving better self-control. (A boy's desire for acknowledgment and status are also valuable assets in getting *him* to accept the responsibilities of the "teacher" role.)

7. Setting an Example

An important way to teach is by example. Parents who are polite, expressive, and sincere teach their sons to speak in the same way. This is not to say that our homes always resound with deeply considered, evocatively expressed statements. At times we all speak too sharply, neglect to explain ourselves, or clam up in a sulk. When we make mistakes, it's important to turn them into teaching opportunities and not to be afraid to apologize. Apologies should be more than the obligatory "I'm sorry." Going further to explain why we're sorry or what consequences we fear might come from our actions or words helps boys put apologies in social perspective. "I'm sorry I snapped at you in the store. Although I truly don't think you need a new video game, a part of me feels bad that I can't afford it right now. I hope I didn't embarrass you."

When we're trying to teach boys to be more socially aware, including the code of social communication, we can find opportunities to provide a positive example at family gatherings, holidays, and so forth. Suppose you're having your extended family over for Thanksgiving. Your sons will see you picking up the house and preparing the dishes, but the meaning of the holiday as a family celebration could get lost unless you articulate some of your thoughts about the social aspects of the gathering. For example, your narrative could be something like "I'm making the green bean casserole the way Aunt Sara always made it for Uncle Troy, because he'll be missing her. Since everyone is so excited to see Frank, I'm putting him in the middle of the table so he can talk to everyone more easily. Grandma is a little sad because her new apartment is too small for all of us, and this is the first year she's coming here; can you think of a way we can make her feel especially welcome?" Such thoughts might be running through your head, but if your sons are old enough not to inadvertently "parrot" you, they can benefit from hearing about the small ways we take care of each other and the consideration for family that motivates our actions. Too often, such discussions are reserved for the girls in our families, if mentioned at all.

If you were to ask me what traits I would most like to see you model for your children, I'd say empathy and honesty. Honesty guides the actions empathy impels, and empathy allows us to be honest in a supportive way.

As we've discussed, it may be helpful to narrate your thoughts by talking out loud in a way that expresses your understanding and appreciation of others. "Sometimes you're quiet in class, but I hope we can find a way to let your teacher know how much you've learned. Do you want to practice with me?" "Sometimes Dad comes home while you're watching your show. I know you don't like to miss a minute, but he looks forward to seeing you and I would like you to remember to say hi and look at him so he knows you see him. If you can do that, I don't mind your watching it and our evening will start out better." "I'm worried that Hannah will think I'm rude for not re-turning her call yesterday, so I'm going to call her up and tell her what happened." Children observe and hear more than most parents realize, and the examples we provide become their template for un-derstanding right and wrong.

During the many psychotherapy sessions in which I've watched parents and children interact, I've come to wonder if we've eroded the distinction between the lives of adults and children far too much. When we talk to our sons in a way that does not respect the bound-aries of that relationship, we render ourselves less effective as teacher or role model. No matter what they might say, or pretend, boys do not want us to be their peers.

While I don't believe we should be authoritarians, sometimes the adventurous and assertive spirit of boys needs to be reined in by someone with a more mature perspective. I was working with a very nice young boy, who had a great sense of humor, in a family session. We were all joking about "Shrek" (a cartoon ogre who likes to eat dis-gusting things like rats and rotten food), and he was getting into a very silly, excitable mood. Soon his teasing of his father ("Would you like some smelly cheese?") began to cross the line ("Dad's feet are so smelly it makes my nose hurt, Dr. Cox!"). Rather than advise his son "That's enough," his father tried to fend off further verbal attacks by changing the subject: "Let's talk about Shrek's donkey! He's a funny one!" Unfortunately, while changing the subject is an effective verbal strategy in some circumstances, this boy's father hadn't preserved enough influence for his suggestion to be heard. When we explain or demonstrate socially correct behavior (in this case, indicating the ex-tent of humor children should use with adults, and that it's not ap-propriate to disclose embarrassing personal information about family members), our sons benefit from our example.

Fathers are under an especially bright spotlight where setting an example is concerned. This is because so many boys are inclined to emulate the behavior and disposition of their fathers. Fathers are boys' primary source of information about what it means to be male. When fathers demonstrate social interest and a social conscience, they are reinforcing an attitude toward others that gives their sons the best chance to be leaders. When fathers are able to demonstrate an ability to be vulnerable (acknowledging mistakes, apologies, ex-pressions of sorrow), at least within the context of their families, they take a giant step toward unburdening their sons of the oppressive male stereotypes associated with stress and social isolation in adult-hood. If you're a father, start this process today.

8. Collaborating

Collaboration is one of the key ingredients of families that run smoothly and with a high degree of cooperation. When our sons observe us collaborating with others, we reinforce the importance of connection. When we show them how we ask for help, compromise, and learn from others, we demonstrate the value of being part of a larger community.

In two-parent families, there is perhaps no more important type of collaboration than that between a child's parents. By collaboration I mean much more than the agreement that may exist when one parent is decidedly dominant with respect to important decisions or choices. When parents actively collaborate, their collective energy revitalizes both their marriage and their parenting alliance and teaches their children the value of mutual respect and empathy.

Before their son was born, Annette and Howard had gotten used to an uneasy peace in which Howard insisted on his way and Annette got around him through wily negotiation and subterfuge. Annette became more directly assertive when it came to their little boy, shutting Howard out of child-rearing decisions almost entirely. By the time Rory was three, she found herself wanting more help with their demanding toddler. In a typical exchange, Howard complained, "She waits until Rory is screaming and then she says, 'Why don't you do something with him?' Then if I try to discipline, she gets mad at me for whatever I say." And Annette replied, "I don't think you understand that he's too young for your kind of discipline. Why don't you learn how to talk to him?" Rory had become verbally aggressive, especially toward Howard, and would cry and throw himself on the floor if Annette reprimanded him for his language. Kids need to see their parents united in a collaborative front, and they need to understand the natural hierarchies in life that give their parents—together when there are two—authority over them. If your relationship is polarized to an extent that collaboration is nearly impossible, even for the sake of your child, then therapy is in order.

The same issues impact nontraditional families. Child rearing is so demanding that most parents seek help from partners, extended family, or friends. Single parents are often particularly in need of respite and support, but negotiating your relationships with the people who are helping you raise your child isn't always easy.

Whether your son has two parents or one, your own parents can be a valuable resource, but these relationships can be particularly tricky. Again, kindness is the key to these collaborative efforts. Your son will learn valuable lessons about empathy and tact if he sees that you value your parents' insights and even tolerate unsolicited advice that may feel intrusive. (Of course, this doesn't mean you should follow advice you feel is inappropriate or ignore caregiving situations that are potentially detrimental to your child.) But when you let your parents know that you're willing to hear their ideas, they may surprise you with how thoughtfully they've considered the issues at hand. If your son is a "chip off the old block," they may have had to address the same issues themselves; they can also remember what problems were resolved naturally, which interventions worked, and how situations evolved over time.

We also need to encourage collaboration in siblings. Older siblings can be taught to help younger siblings. When we confide appropriately in older siblings, we give them a sense of acknowledgment and responsibility. For example, rather than saying to a young boy, "Why can't you be polite like your older brother?" you can ask his older brother if he can help teach his younger brother good ways to greet others or express appreciation. The devil is in the details— collaborating in a way that isn't burdensome or demeaning to either sibling.

Further, we collaborate directly with our children when we involve them in clarifying our goals and expectations. When seeking a behavioral change, it's best to involve them at the outset in establishing the outcome. By asking children to help define those expectations, parents and children have a much better chance of arriving at a common destination. In most cases, boys do best when we discuss behavioral change as a kind of system. Such a framework invites boys to think in a sequential, logical way about how change could take place. In general, when we collaborate, we decrease isolation and make activities more fun. It's simply easier to face challenges of greater complexity when we don't feel alone.

Parents can also be effective collaborators in their relationship with a child's school. Teachers are a great source of information, because they have the advantage of being able to observe your child as an independent social being, away from his family. They have many children, and hours of observation, at their disposal for comparison. It's sometimes difficult us as for parents to reconcile the child we know, as he behaves at home, with the report we receive from school. Yet we are all an amalgam of our different roles, and the public, social role your son adopts in the classroom is important for you to understand. His school training will certainly have an enormous impact on his social and emotional development. Don't hesitate to collaborate with your son's school to understand his public self.

Members of your spiritual community can also help support and guide your child. If you participate in organized religion, the values expressed and shared among your congregation can provide a strong source of affirmation and direction for your child. The experience of joining with others in spiritual practice is very powerful, even though we may come to very different conclusions, and approach our faith in different ways. Peggy, a single mother of a teenage son, related the following: "Ty doesn't usually want to go to church with me. I don't force the issue, but he knows what I get from it and he knows the door is always open. Two months ago, a friend of his was killed in a car accident. He was unreachable. He wouldn't talk about it. Then last week as I was leaving for church he got in the car with me. After the service he asked to speak with our pastor. I don't know what was said, but I'm glad he had a place to go when he needed help." Of course, some people do not belong to a spiritual community in a traditional sense, yet find a sense of the transcendent through experiences such as meditation, art, music or nature, or some other way of subsuming the self-focus and self-absorption that can hinder us. Someone I know described his own beliefs like this: "If there is a God, I feel closest to him in nature; I suppose the forest is my church. When I walk with my kids through the woods, I feel the spirit of communion in the silence, and although we don't always talk, the bonds between us feel stronger." Whether you worship in a cathedral or at the riverbank, or express your spirituality in the age-old rites of your faith or through your dedicated social activism as a secular humanist, introduce your son to your community of faith or service. Although your son may or may not decide to follow your spiritual path, those who share your ideals and values can positively contribute to his social and emotional development.

9. Perseverance

Not everything works the first time you try it. Sometimes it's more important to try longer than it is to try harder. In this sense, perseverance is closely related to the commitment of time—it may take longer than you expect to help your son develop the desired level of social communication skill. The type of daily perseverance required to be an effective parent may be all but invisible to those around you. Yet your ability to persevere can make all the difference in the long run. Janelle, whose son was diagnosed with ADHD, decided to forgo medication and try to work with him on a purely behavioral basis. She would, in essence, have to serve as an external "executive control" system for him, prompting and reminding him to "stay on track" with whatever task he was involved in. "He's nine years old. Yet if I don't remind him before school to say hello to the other kids, he'll run right past them and then be sorry that nobody's talking to him at lunch. I help him keep track of play dates, phone calls, returning games he's borrowed from other kids. Little things, like 'Please stop, turn around and face me when we're talking, or 'We were talking about this; let's finish the subject.' His teachers prompt him in the classroom as well. We have charts, we have a schedule, we have rewards and consequences. What I always try to remember is that there is a limit to what he can do on his own, although I believe he's capable of a lot of improvement. Even if it's the hundredth time I've reminded him of something, I try to ask him nicely and calmly. There have been times when I've had to run around the block a few times because I get so impatient and aggravated. But I know that I'm asking him to do something that is very hard for him, so even if it's frustrating for me, I have to persevere."

Children sometimes begin the process of change long before parents detect it. The seeds of change may first be planted as an idea, a very basic concept that helps a child develop momentum toward a new behavior. When we persevere, we have the best chance of making longer-term gains and building on the seeds of change that have already been planted. When we persevere in teaching and encouraging boys' social development, we make it easier for them to absorb our care and guidance. Change may take months or years to accomplish. But when our sons learn that we won't give up, and that we won't be deterred by their resistance or inability to change quickly, our perseverance is an important element of constancy in their lives.

Boys may feel more secure simply by knowing that our efforts are not subject to the same kind of emotional fluctuation they feel within themselves. Bennett, a painfully shy eleven-year-old, had been encouraged to say hello to every new person he met. "I told him that when he greets another person, he makes them feel recognized, even a little important, and that they are likely to have a good impression of him," said his father. "I take him with me every weekend. I'm an archery salesman, and I go to sporting stores throughout the mid-Atlantic. Bennett rides with me, and we have a pretty good time. When I make a sales call, I introduce him to the store manager or whoever's at the desk. There have been days when he will hardly get out of the truck. He gets a stomachache or something. If it's a rushed day, I admit I can get impatient with that stuff, but when I hear him remembering people's names and smiling, I know we're getting somewhere." Boys appreciate it when they can count on our consistent faith that they will progress.

There are times in a family's life cycle when perseverance becomes extraordinarily important, and adolescence is one of them. During times of rapid change and fluctuation it's more important than ever to persevere so that the longer-term goals and ideals that we hold for our children do not become lost within the everyday conflicts that infiltrate family life. We persevere because we cannot foretell the future. Our perseverance is an expression of faith in our sons that they are worth our effort. By showing boys that we won't give up, that we will meet new problems with renewed creativity, we model an important attitude toward life that our sons will carry into adulthood.

10. Knowing Your Family's Values

Our children need to know what it is that their families stand for. A hundred years ago, it was not uncommon for families in Europe to establish a family creed, and that was an important element that grounded families in a particular mission. I like this notion, because bonding together through shared principle is an important part of making a family a team. Every family needs a compass, and that's the role of a family's core values. We must know these core values because they shape all the other commitments discussed in this chapter. Elements of your core values should be present in how your life expresses the other nine commitments. You'll need to think creatively about how to apply your core values to skills like teaching, collaboration, and modeling.

Take a look at your family's strengths, interests, and expressed values. Where does your moral compass point? Edgar, the owner of a restaurant and catering business, thought of himself as a successful business owner and leader in his community. His wife and son, eighteen-year-old Chase, worked in the restaurant. Edgar said, "We do a good business. One night, my wife and I were sitting at the table, discussing how we could invest some of our profits. We were thinking about opening a second location. We also talked about how much of a bonus we would get and the tax ramifications of paying it all at once or deferring some to the next fiscal year. Chase was at the table, and I like to include him in business discussion because someday it will all be his. I asked his opinion. He thought about it for a moment and asked, 'What about Davey? Do you know why he never smiles?' Davey has been our dishwasher for a few years; he's a bit of a character. I thought Chase was about to tell a joke. Then he said, 'He doesn't smile because he has crappy teeth. He eats soup and soft foods because they hurt him. Maybe we should help him get his teeth fixed, Dad.' " Edgar paused and smiled. "I told him that I paid Davey a competitive wage for his job, that our working conditions were good, and that dental premiums are outrageous. I was thinking to myself that Davey should have finished high school and perhaps have been more personally responsible. I also said we worked hard to build our business and that we deserved some rewards for years of hard work. I talked about the high taxes we pay and the reality that a good business year can be followed by a bad one. Chase just sat there and didn't say anything. I was remembering how idealistic I was at his age, so I said, 'Look, I don't want to put everyone on a health plan, because we just can't do that, but I'll see about helping him out with some dental work. I just can't make any promises, all right?' He just sat there and looked at me. Then finally he said, 'You gave thousands of dollars to the church to build the addition. You walk through the door and everyone treats you with respect and you're proud about that. What's the deal, Dad? Why can't we help the people who are like loyal to us?' In the course of that conversation I went from feeling like a success to a worm in ten minutes, because a part of me knew he was right. He reminded me, it's really easy to talk the talk, but harder to walk the walk. The fact is, our family is in a position to help the people who work for us, at least more than we are. I have to hand it to the kid, he helped refocus family priorities, and I think we all feel better for it."

What are the things that you feel are most essential to helping your son become socially and emotionally strong? Are you living out your intentions? Whether it's being available to help out your neighbors or living in an environmentally responsible manner, living up to the standards you set, on an individual, family, and community level, will bring structure and a moral perspective to your family life.

Putting It All Together

The ten commitments described in this chapter are important considerations for every family, although they will surely be manifest in ways that meet a family's unique needs. Families are scripted over time. Your son's social competence and expressive skills will evolve with the passing years. You'll serve your son's communication needs best when you work on as many levels as possible. I don't expect you to adopt these commitments as some sort of mantra but hope you can think of them as a foundation that will support the specific strategies that follow, strategies you can use to build your son's communication skills and social development for life.

NINE

Leading Boys across the Divide
Building Bridges to Social Communication

■ ■ ■

N ow that you've taken a close look at the psychology of boys and the obstacles they face in crossing the communication divide, you can undoubtedly see how essential it is to nurture the social communication skills they need to lead successful, fulfilling lives. Doing so involves both building the practical skills boys need to become effective communicators and using communication to cultivate your son's social awareness. The strategies described in this chapter can help you prevent communication-related social problems in your son and also minimize their effects when they do occur. You may already be using many of these ideas, in which case you can use this list as a springboard for other approaches to meeting your son's unique needs. The great variety of communication challenges found among boys suggests we need to be flexible and creative. The best approach for one boy may not be the most effective for another. At the same time, some strategies are so fundamental to social and emotional development that most boys' lives will be enhanced by their inclusion in family life.

Building Awareness of Self and Others

Socializing—and I don't mean simply engaging in small talk, but participating fully in the many rich interactions that form the fabric of life for everyone—is all about reciprocity. Your son's early social development (and, in fact, other aspects of his development as well) depends on his building an awareness of himself and others. Such awareness is promoted, in part, through communication. This means you can give your son a boost just by talking with him about himself and others to help him form an identity and distinguish himself from the other people in his world. Although psychologists and child development experts have traditionally thought of this type of differentiation as being a task of early childhood, I believe we can apply these ideas to the social development of older boys as well.

Who Am I?

Self-definition is the critical first step boys must take before they can effectively relate to others. Your son has to develop a definition of himself that goes beyond his physical being, enabling him to recognize himself as a person with individual thoughts and feelings. This can be a slow process, especially for boys more inclined toward physical (kinesthetic) interests than social ones. By adopting ideas like the following, you can help your son become more self-aware and reflective, starting as soon as he is verbal and then continuing throughout his life.

■ *Highlight your son's likes and dislikes.* Notice and comment that he has favorite toys, activities he likes, things that bother him. Asking questions about these things is like holding up a mirror that reveals his mind. Boys who learn to notice what *they* like and dislike are less inclined to be drawn in by the preferences of others. So when your toddler's propensity to state his ideas and preferences in no uncertain (or hushed) terms makes you want to shush him, imagine how helpful this skill will be when you are not available as a surrogate or support—when your son is a teenager trying to decide whether to run for school office even though the other guys think it's uncool, to experiment with drugs at the urging of friends, or to cheat on an exam because "everyone" says you have to get all A's to get into the best colleges.

This is an exercise that builds a "noticing mind"—a mind that can make distinctions, form opinions, build on interests, and appreciate differences. Think of the adults you know who are interesting and informed—my guess is that they have noticing minds. A boy who knows his preferences has more to say than "I dunno" when asked his opinion. And men of many words are those whose opinions ev-eryone *else* wants to hear.

▪ *Allow him to make reasonable choices that fit in with your plans.* Ask him if he'd rather walk to the park or the playground. If you give him the opportunity to make a distinction between two options, his awareness of his preferences will increase. Although parents may in-advertently stress young children with questions that are too open-ended (such as asking a two-year-old "What do you want to do to-day?"), *small* choices engage the will of young boys in an encouraging way. Incidentally, this technique seems to cut down on the frequency of tantrums. You're not only helping your son develop self-awareness; you're giving him a sense of mastery and responsibility.

▪ *Help your son understand his uniqueness within the context of family.* Every child, no matter how young, has a role. When your toddler tags along with you as you do chores, tell him he's your helper. When he does something funny, tell him he made the family smile.

▪ *Ask questions that elicit self-expression.* You don't have to process every emotional experience with your son, but on occasion, stop and help him articulate his feelings. For example, if two brothers are argu-ing over a toy, and one of them feels hurt or angry about the out-come, you might ask, "Are you sad because you didn't get what you wanted? Is it fair that your brother gets to play with your toys some-time? Are you worried you won't get to play with that toy again? What would make you feel happier?" Renowned psychologist Carl Rogers developed a form of therapy where a person's feelings are al-ways acknowledged and articulated. Rogers was perhaps the first psy-chologist to recognize that we all need to be heard and that empath-etic attention can be remarkably healing. In a similar way, asking caring, thoughtful questions of your son will let him know that his feelings count and will help him become sensitive to his emotions. When boys get flustered, and emotions run high, stay calm and do your best to talk through his frustration. The conflict resolution skills you are modeling will become a more natural reflex for boys as they mature.

▪ *Encourage activities that offer opportunity for self-expression.* Let boys dictate letters or e-mails about their day and send them to friends and relatives. Let your son help plan a play date with a friend; he can choose what they'll do or eat. Pretend that he's the daddy and let him pick a stuffed animal to take care of. Have him ask the stuffed animal questions. Let him paint a *sad* or *happy* day, a *silly* cow, an *important* dog.

Who Are You?

Your son's social awareness expands exponentially when he recognizes that others are different from him. This sounds simple, but it's actually an amazing developmental leap. It requires that your son momentarily suspend his own perceptions and consider someone else's reality. Making this leap helps boys appreciate about others that "she (he) is not just another body on earth, but someone with thoughts and feelings that are not the same as mine." Undoubtedly, you encounter adults every day who have not yet reached this stage of development—they're the ones whose needs are always more urgent than yours, who assume you like the same things they like, or give those oddball presents ("Golf shoes? How nice . . .") completely unrelated to your interests. Don't let your son grow up to become one of them.

■ *Encourage inquiry into why other people feel and act the way they do.* If you catch your son watching other people, take the opportunity to get his perspective on what's happening. ("Why is Ryan laughing with Michael?") Help him get comfortable with being asked his opinion. If you ask his opinion about everyday social interaction, he'll turn his attention to it.

■ *Teach your son how to practically consider the thoughts and feelings of others.* "If you make Daddy a birthday card, he'll be pleased." "Sherry hurt her leg; let's cheer her up." "Won't Patty be irritated if you borrow her toys without asking?"

■ *Use engaging metaphors to characterize personal differences.* One fun way you can use a boy's interest in cartoons or action figures is to relate them to everyday aspects of his life. "He was as mad as Mr. MacGregor when Peter Rabbit ate his vegetables!" "What would Superman do in a situation like this?" "Uncle Greg flicked that spider right off! He's as brave as . . ."

Learning How Differences Are Important

As your son develops a solid sense of himself and others, he can begin to explore all the excitement that occurs when different people relate. The important concept here is *context*: What happens when you and I are put together in different circumstances or situations? How does this affect how we feel and behave? This process parallels the ways boys might learn in school. Your fourth grader might discover that if he adds water to baking soda he'll make a paste, but if he adds vinegar he can make a mini-volcano for the science fair. It's all about using combinations thoughtfully and strategically.

■ *Encourage frequent social interaction.* Give your son many opportunities to practice and observe social communication. For younger boys, make playing with other children an important part of their weekly schedule. After a social event (even something as simple as having lunch with a friend or meeting an acquaintance at a store), ask your son about it and make your own observations: "Eddy looked surprised when you said you've been water-skiing" or "I noticed Nigel came with you guys—is he still bossing Jerome around, or is Jerome standing up to him now that he's on the wrestling team?" He will develop "scripts" of increasing complexity and greater insight that inform his future social interactions.

■ *Point out differences between individual interests and mutual interests.* "Both you and your brother like to play trains, but he likes to play soccer and you don't. Sometimes we like the same things, and sometimes we don't." You might observe to your preadolescent son, "I

■ ■ ■

An older client once described his childhood in this way: "My father felt that civilization began to deteriorate as soon as one left Boston or Cambridge. He disliked most people and religions but had a special aversion to unionists and New Yorkers. He died unexpectedly when I was fifteen, and I was sent to live with an uncle in Manhattan. Suddenly I was surrounded by the people my father taught me to dread. I had a deep sense of loyalty to his memory, and so I spent a few years determined to feel that the interesting, kind, and talented people I met were somehow dangerous or inferior. Slowly, and somewhat resentfully, I came to the realization that almost everything he had taught me was wrong, and then I had no idea of how to make amends or reach out to new acquaintances. To this day I have tremendous anxiety meeting people, and I know that people sometimes think of me as a snob. If it weren't for my wife, who has a great interest in others and a talent for conversing with anyone, I'd be lost."

know you don't have much in common with your cousin James, but perhaps you'd like to have him teach you how to fish, and you could show him your fossil collection. Maybe he knows where you could hunt for fossils by the river." Help your son find the bridges and paths that facilitate social connection. Show him by example that as you reach out and associate with people who are different from you, you can find commonalities.

■ *Explain how "likes" go together.* Generally, preferences tend to form in constellations. This is a useful notion for boys to understand, because it helps them make educated guesses about what might appeal to others. For example, if your son's friend likes skateboarding, ice hockey, and tennis, note that he likes physical activities and suggest that it might be thoughtful to buy him a gift certificate to the sporting goods store for his birthday. If your son is planning a sleepover, ask him what his friends will want to do. Talk to him about what your family generally likes to eat and then ask him to suggest what you could plan for tonight's dinner. These kinds of conceptual connections are an important springboard for elements of empathy such as consideration.

■ *Go to places where your son will encounter diversity and differences.* If you live in a homogenous neighborhood, make sure your son has opportunities to know people of other cultures, races, religions, and beliefs. Help him understand that behavior considered polite in some cultures may be rude in others. Reinforce that context shapes interpretation. For example, most eleven-year-old boys are delighted with the notion that it's considered rude *not* to burp after meals in some parts of the world. Wonder out loud if this is because burping acknowledges that the host was able to provide so much food the guest couldn't eat any more. Invite responses and insights.

■ *Use stories and television shows as a jumping-off point to discuss how differences can be complementary.* Choose stories that emphasize cooperation. If your son makes a snide comment about a character, explore what that person may be good at and how his traits could be useful in certain circumstances.

■ *Teach your son about the fun of anticipating what others will think or do.* "How's Mom going to fix those flowers?" "Do you think Charlie will be surprised when he sees your new bike?" Make a big deal of it when boys effectively notice cause and effect. "Justine was worried about you going in her room because she likes things to be very neat, but you were careful, and now she doesn't worry about you going in her room anymore." Encourage your son to anticipate how other people will react to his actions and choices.

■ *Teach your son to disagree agreeably.* Teach him that it's okay if people don't agree all the time. Small children sometimes need to be reassured that people can still be friends and like each other with a difference of opinion. Explain the difference between being "mean" and disagreeing. Older children need to learn how to state their differences without dismissing the value of the other person's perspective. "I know you're angry at Jim for what he said, but maybe he has a right to be angry at Coach. What would you have done in that situation?"

Life's Cast of Characters

As your son begins to understand how people react individually to circumstances and how they differ in their thoughts and feelings, he can also begin to relate how people are similar. You may have noticed that older people aren't typically too surprised by others. That's because over time they've been exposed to many different types of people, and they can see aspects of those people in the new people they meet. They have a reference point for making an educated guess about what a person is like, at least until direct observation proves otherwise. This kind of knowledge is relative to one's stage of development. You might know a savvy fourteen-year-old who notices that his new friend is bragging a lot. It may remind him of a friend he had in seventh grade who he found out was a big-time exaggerator. Consequently, he's a little more skeptical when new peers make extraordinary statements about themselves.

As children learn to make distinctions, they develop the ability to categorize behavior and ways of thinking. This is a useful skill in learning to judge character and in knowing how to relate effectively to different kinds of people. Someone who does not learn from past experiences or cannot relate the traits of one person to another loses an important social advantage. What we as parents might assume will develop through intuition may need to be taught in a more pragmatic way to many boys.

■ *Relate important people in your son's life to characters in books and television.* Literature and the arts provide wonderful opportunities to learn about human character. Compare the personality traits of fictional characters with those of real people. By extension, rely on the problem-solving skills of characters depicted in books or television as a template to help your son think through social and emotional challenges.

- *Ask your son about how his friends are similar and different.* Note that he can "group" his friends in all kinds of combinations—friends who like jokes, friends who are good athletes, friends who like computer games. "How come those guys always play together?" asks him to observe what people have in common.

- *Discuss how circumstances can alter a person's character or behavior.* This is important, because although categorization is a useful lens through which to view people, we should not be restricted by a limited picture of someone. "She was quiet, but that job gave her a lot of confidence. Now she's more outgoing." "Tom doesn't mean to be cranky, but he's had a toothache for days."

- *Ask what types of people your son likes for friends.* Does he like people who share his interests or who are interesting because they are different? Does he like people who behave in a certain way? Why?

Natural Hierarchies

As your son identifies the individuals who fill his life, he can begin to understand the interactions of groups and the formation of social hierarchies. An important aspect of understanding and accepting hierarchies is recognizing how they occur naturally through basic social structures like family, school, and teams. The starting point for developing this awareness is always with parent–child relationships and the requirement that children respect parental authority. This doesn't mean your son should stand at attention and spring to your every command like an obedient dog! It should mean that your son recognizes you have the final say in important matters and will make decisions regarding his well-being. There's nothing more difficult than trying to regain authority once you've lost it or to establish parental control when you've never had it. And it's easy to let all the little opportunities to establish natural hierarchies slide, giving boys too much power to call the shots. As children push boundaries further and further (hoping somebody will set a limit), the return to reasonable behavior takes longer. In my practice, I call this the "dictator syndrome." Dictators become infatuated with power and often seek to leverage their power for power's sake. The result is social chaos, with every interaction marked by manipulation. I want to emphasize that establishing yourself as an authority figure does not mean yelling, punishment, or rigidity. True leadership allows you to consistently treat your son with love and compassion and interpret obstacles as problems that have yet to be solved rather than expressions of oppositionality or defiance. Most important, an effective leader clearly supports and articulates, through words and deeds, the values of the family.

When a boy understands and respects natural hierarchies and modifies his behavior according to circumstances, he's taking his first steps toward accepting the social contract that binds individuals together. Of course, our intent is not to foster thoughtless submission to authority. But we should be working toward raising boys who can balance self-interests with the needs and rules of larger groups. Some ways to heighten awareness of natural hierarchies include:

■ *Ask your son to notice how people can change roles.* Comment that his teacher likes to ride his motorcycle on his days off or that Aunt Barbara used to be a "hippie." Mention that it's okay to call a neighbor by his first name unless you're at football practice, where he should always be referred to as "Coach."

■ *Teach your son that behavior changes according to circumstances.* Circumstances can include the places we are ("We don't shout in the hospital because sick people need to rest"), the others we are with ("Even though it's okay to tease your friends, Grandma doesn't understand that you're only joking"), and the urgency of the situation ("It's okay that you interrupted Dad on the phone when Brendan got hurt").

■ *Explore the reasons for hierarchies.* "What would happen if there was a big fire and there was no fire chief?" With an older son you can discuss why societies value elders or the practical reasons for teachers being in charge of a classroom.

■ *Explore appropriate avenues for protest.* "If you think the school's rule about no cell phones is wrong, what if all the kids wrote letters asking the principal to change the rule and listed good reasons for allowing them?"

■ *Give him opportunities to lead.* It's not so difficult to respect authority when you have a chance to exercise some command yourself. For a young child, it might be putting him in charge of making sure the family doesn't feed the dog too many treats each day, so the dog doesn't get sick. A favorite technique of mine in working with boys who have behavior problems in school is to put them in charge of coaching younger boys with behavior problems. Teaching something to others is a fantastic way to learn.

■ *Help boys understand that privileges often come with responsibilities.* "I wish I could go with you guys, but when I agreed to be a volunteer fireman, I knew I would occasionally have to work on Sunday." "If you're going to be a crossing guard, you have to get up earlier than other kids—they're counting on you."

■ *Minimize commands.* It's important to let your son know where you stand, but if you march around constantly giving orders, he'll feel weak, humiliated, or angry. Decide which ground rules are important to you and offer choices or compromise when you can. Notice and reward compliance and positive behavior whenever possible. The times when you issue a "command" should be so rare and surprising that your son understands the situation is urgent and responds accordingly.

■ *Don't be apologetic about making the decisions.* I believe families should operate on democratic principles, considering the perspectives and needs of everyone, but with a clear understanding that parents are in charge of establishing the rules that govern family behavior. Practically speaking, every interaction with your son can't turn into a long debate or reinforce the illusion that his judgment is as sound as your own. At the same time, the way your son develops good judgment himself is by hearing you verbalize your reasons for making the decisions you do.

Story Time

For young children, stories are the window to a world larger than their immediate environment. Through stories children expand their awareness of different people and places and, in turn, their understanding of their own realities and potentials. Unfortunately, as many boys get older their interest in stories diminishes. You can help keep that interest alive by discussing books and making storytelling a family tradition.

Another important aspect of storytelling is that it provides children with a sense of narrative—things happen in sequences; there's cause and effect; actions converge. We learn stories by heart: fostering this sensitivity to narrative helps boys meaningfully know the pace, rhythm, and reasons of life's interactions.

■ *Read together.* There's probably no better way to develop your son's reading ability (phonological awareness, vocabulary) and social communication skills than establishing reading as an important activity in your home. Read to young children daily and make it fun—snuggle up, use silly voices, let your son pick out books and get his own library card. Encourage your teenage son to read books about his interests. When possible, read those books yourself so you can talk to him insightfully about what he has read. Parents often complain about how detached adolescent boys can be, yet collective reading provides a much less self-conscious way to explore feelings and thoughts.

■ *Help your son try on roles.* Encourage his imaginative projection as a character. "I'm a helicopter! You're a jet!" Getting down on the floor and entering his make-believe world encourages play that helps him explore different roles imaginatively. (It's amazing how much more your son will tell you if you ask him a question in a silly voice with a sock puppet on your hand.) Older children can explore roles through performance—acting, singing, or dancing, or, if they prefer, playwriting, songwriting, and choreography. For adolescents disinclined toward these types of activity, you may have to be creative. Perhaps your son won't take acting classes but will play charades or a board game that requires nonverbal clues. Perhaps he won't make up a story for you, but he might for a young child who's visiting. A karaoke machine or a long, boring car ride may provide the motivation to sing with you.

■ *When making up stories for your son, come to an exciting point in the narrative and ask him to provide the next line.* You can build whole stories by trading lines. (Mom: It was a dark and stormy night. Son: A boy named Iggy had to find a treasure. Mom: . . .) Kids are very forgiving if you aren't the best storyteller and will learn a lot by helping you piece together a story. This is a great activity for a long car ride.

■ *Write letters.* Establish this as a habit early on—have your child help write invitations to parties and special events, send holiday cards, notes to relatives who live far away, and thank-you letters. Make it fun and don't be rigid about the form or the length of his communication. A box of blank cards with some cool stickers and

■ ■ ■

When her son started having problems at school, rather than lecture, a friend of mine chose to tell him bedtime stories about a boy named Carlos. Carlos faced difficulties that were similar to her son's problems—and during the stories, through trial and error, he tried different solutions, some silly, some quite effective. Her son began interjecting his own story lines for "Carlos stories"—first as problems Carlos would face, but later solutions Carlos could use, too. "We told Carlos stories incessantly for about six months," she said. "But as things smoothed out in his class, he asked for the stories less often. Every now and then he asks for a Carlos story, but it's more like he wants to visit an old friend than needing the stories to help with a specific problem. He's developed his own problem-solving skills well enough now."

markers will help. Enlist your friends and relatives to reply by mail to your son. Letter writing encourages more deliberation about word choices than phone calls and is a skill that will help your son when he starts to send e-mail.

Feeling and Thinking

Learning is almost always enhanced by emotion, because emotion stimulates our perceptual awareness, allowing us to sense and absorb information on multiple levels. It's important to help boys recognize how to learn through both cognitive and emotional pathways. And the very first emotions your son needs to recognize are his own.

■ *Help your son distinguish thoughts from feelings.* We can think about things in one way but feel another way altogether. Boys who are inclined to be systematizers may tamp out their feelings under the heavy foot of logic and facts. Doing so, they lose a powerful way of knowing and relating to others. If you sense that your son is sweeping his feelings under the rug or intellectualizing, let him know that it's okay to show his feelings. For example, if your son says, "Marc was made captain of the team. It makes sense that he got elected because he has the highest batting average," you could begin your conversation by saying, "I noticed that you looked sad when you said that. Even though he may be the best athlete, maybe he's not the best at bringing the team together. Since you're such a dedicated player, I wonder if you feel disappointed that you weren't considered?"

■ *Reinforce that feelings don't have to be justified.* We all feel excited, angry, sad, happy, frustrated, jealous, proud, or vindictive at times. Sometimes we might feel this way "for no good reason." But rather than asking boys not to feel a certain way, try to limit your corrections to false interpretations or assumptions. In other words, if your son is envious of his brother, you might contradict his erroneous *impression* that you love his brother more, or you might let him know he cannot act on his jealousy and pinch his brother. But rather than saying, "Don't feel that way," perhaps you can acknowledge his envy or even talk about a time that you felt envious too.

■ *Role-play people and animals with an emphasis on emotion.* This is an expedient way to grow your son's emotional vocabulary. For example, using a puppet, you could say "Elephant is *frustrated* because he keeps on forgetting where he left his peanuts." Have the elephant puppet mumble, "I'm so frustrated . . . where are they?" and bumble as he searches through your son's toy box, under his baby blanket, and other silly places, looking ever more frantically. As your son giggles, he'll learn what "frustrated" means. He'll also have fun hiding the peanuts. Older boys might appreciate your satiric reinterpretation of an everyday event, especially if you can be humorously self-deprecating. "And so, determined to get his attention and dazzle him with my penetrating, incisive wit, I told my best joke and messed up the punch line."

■ *Allow your son to explore a range of emotional responses to the same situation.* Ask him hypothetical questions: "What if a monster ate your sister's toys?" "Would you be more excited or nervous if you got to meet the president?" "When Kevin won at arm wrestling, was he feeling happy about being so strong or worried about beating his father?"

Language and Communication Skills

Learning to differentiate between oneself and others is helped by increasing familiarity with words, language, and interpersonal communication. Boys gain this familiarity in several important ways, all of which parents can promote through practice and insight.

Reading

As Chapter 7 discussed, reading promotes verbal dexterity and intellectual development that will directly translate to social and academic success in life.

■ *Make reading a family priority.* Sit close to your young son so he associates your physical warmth, the crinkle of the turning page, and the musty smell of a well-loved book with the pleasure of reading. Make sure all caregivers in the family participate in reading to boys too.

■ *Make your home reader friendly.* Fill your home with reading materials; let your son see you reading; make sure there's a quiet, comfortable spot for him to read; and avoid being unreasonably picky or judgmental about what he reads.

> **■ ■ ■**
> **Money talks . . .**
> Dollar for dollar, do you spend as much on books for your son as you spend on videos and computer games? An intellectually impoverished home has a tower of DVDs and no bookshelf.

■ *Encourage leisure reading that is action and emotion oriented.* Even though you won't choose all your son's books, encourage those with strong narrative story lines, social interaction, and a range of emotions.

Climbing the Language Ladder

Once boys develop a basic vocabulary, help them use it. There are boys with a relatively smaller fund of words at their command who are excellent communicators because they understand the meaning of those words precisely and can use them creatively and flexibly. This type of expressive depth is at least as important as having expressive breadth—knowing a great many words. And as boys deposit words in their vocabulary banks, they can use them to understand and acquire more words.

■ *Build on word understanding.* Use a word your son knows to help him learn similar words. For example, if it's raining and your son says, "It's a sad day," you could agree: "Yes, it's a sad, dreary, depressing day." If he knows the word *emergency,* you could suggest he drive his super rescue car "to take care of that emergency and that other disaster over there too." We should work toward giving boys adequate descriptive tools to make their thoughts known.

■ *Help your son distinguish between similar word choices.* Be specific in your own word usage, and if you're prone to expressive superlatives ("I'm frantic!" "It's awesome!"), be sure to give your son some more nuanced choices ("No, I'm not furious, but I sure am irritated.")

■ *Talk to your son about how context shapes perception and meaning.* A boy telling his father he got four A's on his report card might be perceived differently if he tells him when his father discovers a window broken by a baseball ("Sorry, but I'm not all bad"), when his father is boasting about his brother's pitching ("I'm great too"), or when his father has had a difficult day ("Cheer up, Dad!").

Word Play

If play is the work of children, word play should be where children work on developing the language skills that enrich life.

■ *Play word games.* Sing, make up rhymes, give your son a cool nickname, invent and define nonsense words, do puzzles, use pretend accents, play Scrabble, make terrible puns. The more verbally dexterous and interesting you are, the more likely your son is to notice and develop those skills himself.

■ *Sing.* Songs are poems set to music. Teach your baby lots of songs and he'll learn lots of words. He'll develop his memory and awareness of phonemes too. I've found that older boys never lose their interest in learning new things from music, which is why I often use it in therapy.

■ *Teach your son how to tell a joke.* And when he tries to tell you a joke, laugh.

■ *Encourage interest in other languages.* If you speak another language in the home, consider using that language for especially important or interesting communications.

> ■ ■ ■
>
> The cookie jar password: Boys can be allowed another cookie if they can tell you a synonym ("What's another word for big?" "Huge!" "Very good—a huge cookie for you!"), a word that rhymes ("What rhymes with jiggle?"), or make up a definition to a nonsense word ("What would a grizzlebot be?").

Noticing Aloud

You may be able to figure out a computer program or build a boat by looking at a manual, but it's a lot easier if someone just explains and shows you how to do it. In the same way, we can save our sons a lot of confusion, heighten their interest in social communication, and prevent them from blocking out domains of life that just seem inscrutable by actively describing events and serving as their "translators." Boys who tend to perceive things inaccurately, because they're intensely self-conscious or prone to attributing the wrong intent to others, will benefit from your guided tour of language and life.

Noticing your son's communication skills out loud may feel awkward to you at first, but it's important. Not only does it ensure that he learns these social communication skills, but it also demonstrates that this is an important aspect of who he is and that you're invested in his success. Explaining your choices helps him break the code of social communication.

■ *Think aloud during problem solving.* Your son will begin to understand how you run through the steps, from defining the problem to considering possible solutions and choosing an acceptable response. If you talk about solving a social problem that involves communication ("How will I turn down the job without hurting Uncle Joe's feelings?"), so much the better.

■ *Practice identifying other people's emotions.* Ask your son simple questions, such as, "How did Jack feel when you asked him if you could postpone your lunch together? How do you know that? How did he look? What did he say?" Sometimes boys are reluctant to engage in such conversations. If he perseveres and puts some thought into his answers, make sure you praise him for his insights. If he tries to respond but can't, give him helpful prompts.

■ *Provide public praise for your son's good use of expressive skills.* Public praise doesn't mean getting out your megaphone in the town square, but it does mean expressing your admiration out loud, either just to him or in front of his family or friends if it won't embarrass him too much. "You were polite to Mrs. Walker and answered her questions in a very friendly way. I was proud of you."

■ *Notice how others use words.* "Bill tends to exaggerate when he's excited." "Sharon sometimes repeats herself when she's nervous."

"Notice how every time Steve tried to join the conversation, Joey cut in with another story about skiing?" "Sean is such an optimist that if someone stole his bike, he'd probably only want to talk about how excited he was about the possibility of getting a new one." "When you hear Pastor Paul talk about his work in the clinic, it's inspirational because you know he puts his whole heart into his mission." If your son is a literalist and he's missing the irony in his friends' conversation, mention it to him. "I don't think Dustin really liked camp. In fact, I think he meant the opposite. Did you notice his expression and tone of voice?"

▪ *Discuss multiple perspectives of the same situation.* Help your son understand that people may understand events, perceive actions, or hear words very differently. Encourage him to openly discuss possible interpretations with you. Destigmatize the need to query others about what someone meant or what something means.

Nonverbal Communication

Body language can speak for itself or, when used in conjunction with words, confirm, intensify, or deny verbal messages. Boys who unintentionally convey negative meanings through their nonverbal communication suffer undeserved consequences.

As discussed in Chapter 7, pragmatic communication involves learning to use social codes and conventions. This type of learning doesn't always come easily but is helped substantially by compassionate parental coaching.

▪ *Role-play pragmatic communication skills.* "Try using your voice to show interest in getting to know me." Talk to your son about how he can handle situations he encounters at home and school. "If you want to join the circle, wait until there's a gap between two kids rather than pushing." "Let's try saying hello to each other again, using just our eyes."

▪ *Integrate gestures with words.* Show your son by example how nonverbal expression can mimic words. Playing charades could be a good choice for stiff or stoic boys.

▪ *Reinforce the power of smiling.* Rather than commanding "Smile!" wait until your son does smile in a friendly way and praise him afterward. Have your adolescent son conduct an experiment where he keeps track of how people respond to him on a day when he smiles at everyone, as compared with a day when he rarely smiles. Analytically inclined boys may be more easily convinced by this type of data.

Interpersonal Skills

Starting when he is at a young age, help your son become adept at interacting with others. A boy with good interpersonal skills is aware of his own thoughts and feelings and knows that others have distinct and different thoughts and feelings. He can apply his understanding of both to read how he's perceived by others and regulate his words and actions. In contrast, boys with poor interpersonal skills tend to be unaware of their own feelings, have difficulty reading others, don't know how others see them, or have difficulty modifying their words or actions according to the circumstances. Haven't you heard boys described like this? "He just doesn't realize how he comes off"; "He doesn't know when enough's enough!"; or "Couldn't he tell it was the wrong time to say that?"

■ *Practice greetings and good-byes.* It helps to prepare young boys for introductions and departures if you practice at home ahead of time. Positive reinforcement, through praise for a job well done, is much more effective than on-the-spot requests or demands.

■ *Teach your son how to give compliments.* When he says something nice to you, tell him how happy it makes you feel. Ask him to comment positively on other students in school or peers in the neighborhood. If he says he doesn't know how, give him several examples and model the giving of compliments at home.

■ *Provide guidance about making conversational transitions.* Help your son understand the necessary give-and-take of conversation and how to transition from discussing his own interests to inquiring about something of interest to another person. Doing so reinforces that conversation is inherently social.

■ *Encourage boys to relate cause and effect.* Storytelling and reading help boys develop a theoretical understanding of cause and effect. Be sure to help your son apply those lessons by pointing out how his actions have caused reactions in his own life: "By bringing out the Monopoly game you helped prevent a fight between your sisters and kept everyone occupied. Nice job."

Consistent Reinforcement

For boys who find communication challenging or uninteresting, your consistent reinforcement and creative energy are key. Remember, you're fighting to give your son a chance to participate fully in his society. If he required daily physical therapy to walk, you'd provide it. If he needs daily reinforcement to talk, you're going to do that too, right?

■ *Provide feedback about prosody.* Let your son hear how he sounds. "I don't think you realize that you sound bored about going to see a movie with Angela. I wonder how that's making her feel about going?" How we say words (prosody) greatly impacts meaning. If you have a talent for acting or mimicry, provide your son with an opportunity to see and hear what his communication feels like. Objectively ask him: how does he think he sounds?

■ *Encourage boys to elaborate their description of their feelings.* If your son says he's "bummed out," ask if he's disappointed, annoyed, or angry at himself. If your son hesitates to talk about his emotions, he may be avoiding the discomfort of dealing with them, or he may genuinely not be able to define them. Finding out can take a lot of patience and detective work on a parent's part. Consider enlisting the help of a trusted friend or therapist if necessary.

■ *Praise him for self-disclosure and process-oriented thinking.* Pay attention to what he does well in the line of communication and be sure to notice his successes. Make praise even more meaningful by explaining why or how self-disclosure was helpful. Reciprocate by modeling appropriate self-disclosures, reinforcing that difficult feelings, mistakes, and periodic anxieties are a part of all phases of life.

Emphasize Natural Interests

You can encourage your son to be more verbal and socially adept if you capitalize on his interests, whether it's a particular book or character, sport, game, or hobby. Open the door to conversation. If talking about feelings and emotions is beyond him at this moment, try building up your relationship by conversing about something he's interested in. By establishing that you're interested in what he's interested in, you're communicating care and concern.

■ *Relate his interest to other life situations.* For example, if he plays a sport, notice how the team dynamics compare with a political race. "Not only do you want to win the game; your team especially wants to beat those guys because you think they're cheaters. That's why Erin's mom is running for city council and really wants to win—she thinks the people who are on the council now have been dishonest."

■ *Use his excitement.* If your son really relishes a band, dirt bike racing, Jimmy Neutron, or chess, foster his excitement to expand his emotional range. "You're really excited about going to the concert— wouldn't you love to be in the band? Can you imagine the feeling of being on national television? I wonder how people handle the pressure of a big tournament." Sometimes it's easier to jump-start your son's interest in discussing feelings when you focus on his idols.

Strong Minds, Hearts, and Spirits

When we talk about making boys strong, we use the term in a variety ways. We want boys to be physically healthy and emotionally capable. And we want them to lead their lives and interact with others in ways that are good, helpful, brave, and steadfast, even in the face of adversity. We generally fasten these life skills together under the rubric "character" and try our level best to develop a good one in our sons. Yet talking about the character development and moral education of boys may unfortunately sound like a quaint or even antiquated notion. Such a focus may be associated with authoritarianism and narrow-minded prescriptive policies of the past. In this country, especially, we tend to be highly suspicious of any institution— educational, community, or political—that makes value judgments about what's good and right and proposes to instill those values in our children. We like to have the freedom to choose for ourselves what's best for our sons.

By the same token, our society and our children pay a high price when we as parents are unwilling or unable to give boys a viable roadmap to responsible adulthood. Children don't grow up in a vacuum, and if we don't provide them with some guidance, they look to the culture at large—the street, popular entertainment, or whatever compelling influences (good or bad) that are presented to them. Perhaps ironically, many of us who don't want others to dictate what's right for our sons feel strongly that other people's sons need intervention. That's one reason our society tends to have a rather incoherent pastiche of social programs and a lively, ongoing debate about the role of community in shaping our youth. You can't be a responsible parent without engaging in that debate and knowing where you stand with respect to your son's social and emotional needs.

I strongly believe that boys who are able to care for others and express themselves are much more likely to be happy and successful. These traits grow from the common roots of self-esteem and self-confidence. These capabilities are enabled by the encouragement and opportunity for practice provided by parents. When boys have a working awareness of their own feelings and some insight about the motivations of others, they can make choices about how to use that knowledge to act and express themselves. While self-interested action is not necessarily incompatible with the greater good, a boy's social conscience helps him mediate the psychological tension between those perspectives. The lives of boys are filled with scenarios that play out this drama on a daily basis; sibling rivalries, conflicts on the playground, arguments with coaches and teammates, and frustration with family rules are but a few examples of how boys struggle to balance their personal wants and needs with those of larger groups. Helping your son develop a strong and healthy character gives him the best chance of finding happiness in the balance of individual and group needs that life requires and increases the likelihood that he will be appreciated by his immediate family, future spouse or children, and community.

Practicing Empathy

As we've discussed, empathy requires us to experience the feelings of others and in some cases to take appropriate action. A boy with sympathy notices when a friend is embarrassed, but a boy with empathy tells a joke about the time he went "brain dead" in the middle of a speech to make his friend laugh and feel better.

■ *Encourage identification with other people's feelings.* "Katie's been studying for that exam for months. Don't you think she's relieved she's finally passed?" "You're like your dad—you get embarrassed when people praise you a lot."

Help your son understand how his words and actions impact others. "Do you think it hurt Elias's feelings when you laughed at his photo?" If a friend or family member is sad or unwell, ask him how he could cheer that person up. If your son makes you proud or happy, tell him why.

■ *Verbalize approval of good character traits.* Take the opportunity to notice when your son is being thoughtful, kind, honest, considerate, responsible, friendly, outgoing, insightful, mature, reliable, persever-ant, sympathetic, hardworking, funny, brave, helpful, cheerful, care-ful, appropriate, sociable, attentive, or consistent.

■ *Make your praise specific to the action.* "You're really responsible when it comes to taking care of the dog" is better than "You're a good boy," in that it fastens the praise to a precipitating behavior. Some parents give their sons constant, generalized praise in an attempt to convince them the statement is true, as an unthinking habit or as a way of building self-esteem. It's better to inform your son about what he's doing that makes him "good." Children can separate "feel good" chatter from a well-placed, attentive compliment. (It's the difference between your boss's saying, "Great job, great job, everybody," and her saying, "Steven, nobody else had your insight about how we could cross-market the account, and it made us look brilliant!")

■ *Emphasize the importance of acting on feelings of empathy.* "If Douglas is feeling left out, why don't you invite him over?" "If you're worried about Sarah, give her a call and let her know she has your vote."

People Come First

Boys who tend to be fascinated by their interior world, who have difficulty appreciating or understanding others, or who are highly self-conscious can constrict their social experience to the point that it stunts their ability to form meaningful relationships with others. Helping your son move from self-absorption to involvement with others at a young age will save him from rejection and isolation as an adult.

■ *Verbally explore the value of friendships.* Talk about the things you can learn from a friend and how friends support and help each other.

■ *Introduce your son to friendly people.* When your son is taking his first steps into the social realm, arrange for him to be around adults who are good with children and children who are kind and well be-haved. Note what kind of people your son responds to. A boisterous, gregarious person, while well intentioned, may not be the best match for your son.

■ *Emphasize that other people are what make life fun and interesting.* "Howard's coming to visit! He knows some really cool magic tricks—maybe he'll show you!"

■ *Model social interest within your own home.* Planning parties, visiting neighbors, and playing games with others all provide object lessons in the value of sociability. Busy parents with children often feel short of time and the energy needed for company. But if you're always avoiding, complaining about, or fighting with your family and associates, maybe you haven't made a compelling case for socialization.

> ■ ■ ■
> ## The Power of Association
> If your son has an activity that he particularly likes (playing on the slides at the playground or visiting the zoo, for example), make sure you always invite a playmate along so that he begins to associate "fun" with the company of others.

Stressing Love and Compassion

Obviously, I don't have to tell you to love your son and treat him compassionately. But social pressures to make sure boys grow up to be strong men who can hold their own in a tough world can creep into the way we demonstrate our love for our sons. Too often boys end up denied the physical demonstrations of affection that are doled out liberally to girls. Fathers especially may be too inclined to suppress hugs and kisses in favor of the rare pat on the back. Or they simply don't say "I love you" very freely. Holding back on expressions of love and compassion for our sons is tantamount to starving them emotionally. And leaving the greater part of emotional caretaking to mothers sends a very damaging message to our sons.

■ *Talk about love.* Not all love is romantic love, and many people mistake sexual attraction for love. Especially as your son gets older, discuss different ways love is expressed and experienced. This is particularly important for hormonally charged adolescents.

■ *Talk about why people live in families.* Converse about the joys, rewards, compromises, and challenges of family life. If you're fortunate enough to be in a happy marriage or partnership, talk about the things that make your relationship a success. If you're divorced, try to find something positive to say about your former spouse and try to find ways for your son to have a healthy relationship with his other parent. If you're single by choice, don't speak disparagingly of marriage in blanket terms; it may be a good option for your son in the future.

■ *Help your son treat girls with respect.* Ask your son what traits he would look for in an ideal partner. Make sure he recognizes and acknowledges the humanity of the girls he socializes with. This can be difficult if there's a misogynistic boy running his peer group or if he is unduly influenced by popular culture. By the same token, boys can be goaded into dating and sex prematurely by peer pressure or sexually aggressive girls. Help your son expand his definition of masculinity beyond sexual activity and help him develop some face-saving responses if he's being swarmed by phone calls and come-ons before he's ready.

Cultivating a Conscience

We make sure boys develop their physical skills through practice and exercise and their academic skills through lessons and homework. Relying on a similar approach, we can effectively cultivate a boy's conscience in a thoughtful, cumulative manner. Conscience is a compass that will navigate your son safely through muddy moral situations and foggy social conditions. A boy who has been led to develop his own conscience will have more to say, and more courage to say it when it really counts. Conscience helps us find our way through difficult choices and prompts our compassion for others— even when it's hard to do.

■ *Discuss the difference between doing the "right" thing and what you want to do.* "I know you want to skip Terry's party to go to Alec's, but you would hurt Terry's feelings, and you promised him you'd be there."

■ *Introduce your son to the concept of personal ethics.* "Porter didn't accept the reward for returning the wallet he found, since he would have done it anyway." "Your father and I disagree about the death penalty, because . . ." Ask your son what he would do in difficult situations: "What if you saw a starving man steal some food?" "What if he was stealing the food from a king who hoarded all the people's food? What if he stole it from a hungry child? What if you could be thrown in jail for not reporting him?"

■ *Self-disclose about difficult choices and their consequences in your own life.* It can be helpful to talk about your own moral struggles, especially when your son is having a problem. "When I was your age, I really loved candy, and once I took a piece from the store without paying for it, too. I knew it was wrong, but I was mad because my sister had been given a candy bar for good grades, but not me. My mom made me give it back, and I had to apologize to the store owner." Life's hardest lessons are learned a little more easily when we realize we haven't learned them alone.

Community Involvement

We live in a world of distorted proportions. The tragedies suffered by people on the other side of the world come right into our homes through TV and the Internet and can make us feel despair for those thousands of miles away but helpless to make things right. At the same time, too often we don't even know our next-door neighbors' names. Yet the value of living in a community is the opportunity to know others, to help and be helped as needed. However you define your community—through proximity, common interest, or other bond—the best way to introduce your son to that community is to let him roll up his sleeves and get involved. A boy's involvement in community helps put his life in perspective and connect with others beyond the more intimate realms of family and close friends. Some ways to introduce your son to his community include:

■ *Explore how compassion can be translated into action.* Ask your son how he thinks your family can help others, and follow through with his suggestions if possible.

■ *Demonstrate a family commitment to community organizations.* If your son sees you volunteering at his school, running in a 5K charity race, donating blood, or attending a rally, he'll notice that your life isn't circumscribed solely by home and work—that you're part of a larger constellation of relationships.

■ *Expand his world.* Ally yourself with your son in fulfilling an important social goal. Capitalize on his natural interests. If your son loves animals, you can talk to him about the plight of strays and volunteer for the humane society together. If he's a computer wizard, have him set up a website for a local charity or coach senior citizens in getting online. In some situations, just a willingness to help makes you a hero—and assists boys in internalizing a self-image of being a helpful person. For some boys, it can be very liberating to have an important role outside home or school, especially if they are not feeling very successful in those domains.

■ *Talk about the community in front of your children.* Talk about what's happening at your son's school, the next presidential campaign, or why the local land conservancy bought a nearby farm. Your son may resist talking to you about how he's feeling or what he's doing, but may be more verbal when you ask him his opinions. A contrary boy may enjoy the opportunity to spar with you over more controversial topics, and as long as the conversation is basically respectful, you can use the debate as an opportunity to strengthen his critical thinking skills and verbal dexterity.

Putting Competition into Perspective

As we've discussed, many boys tend to be at their most confident and expressive in competitive settings. Of course, other boys shut down in competitive situations—especially when they don't fare well in comparison with peers. But competition is a fact of life, and there are a lot of strings attached to it for boys. For better or worse, much of our sense of accomplishment and self-definition occurs in counterpoint to others. Helping your son learn to deal with competition can make a big difference to his expressive and social skills.

■ *Put competition into perspective.* The best time to do this is before the competition, so your remarks carry weight whether your son wins or loses.

■ *Beware of mixed messages.* A coach who says "winning isn't everything" but never lets less talented kids play contradicts his own words.

■ *Teach your son to be a gracious winner and loser.* The former promotes empathy; the latter promotes emotional self-control and self-worth.

■ *Beware of living vicariously.* Boys are very sensitive to their parents', and, I'm afraid, mostly their fathers', desires for them. Some boys will virtually knock themselves out trying to please. Most often we think of boys who try to fulfill their fathers' dreams on the sports field. In my clinical work, I have seen a similar phenomenon among boys who feel compelled to prove themselves as exceptionally creative, clever, popular, or intellectual to please a parent. Any of these pressures is a heavy burden to bear and can have long-term, intergenerational effects.

Encouraging Experimentation

All the skills and traits that strengthen boys' social communication can be developed through practice and exposure. Our job as parents and mentors is to facilitate as broad a variety of situations as possible where boys get the opportunity to acquire and build on these talents.

Encouragement

Just as your son might require a reminder to practice for his piano lesson, need assistance with a school project, or learn from you how to throw a ball, teaching boys to become social and communicative requires parental encouragement. Help minimize the risks of social experimentation by suggesting practical strategies for specific situations: "I bet more kids in your class would talk to you if you let them know you're interested in them." "Maybe you could ask Julia out to lunch before you ask her if she wants to be your date for the prom."

■ *Help your son initiate social activities.* Help him plan and host a party at your house or start a club. A young boy who likes racing cars can have the neighborhood kids come to a "car rally" in your backyard dirt pile. You can offer to drive and supervise your preteen and his friends at a concert. If you normally have an annual holiday party, suggest that your teenager "piggyback" on the party by inviting his friends too—perhaps provide a separate space for them to congregate.

■ *Encourage him to issue invitations.* If he wants you to take him somewhere, ask him to invite a friend: "Wouldn't it be fun if you brought Bret with us when we go to the lake?" "Since we're running up to the mall, why don't we invite Skylar?"

■ *Stimulate social curiosity through travel and new experiences.* Kids can be provincial or in a rut, just like adults. Expand your son's horizons. If his environment is stimulating and experiences are exciting, he'll have a greater need and desire to communicate.

■ *Encourage new friendships.* As a general principle, you'll be letting your son observe and respond to a wide range of human expression. In a smaller sense, if he has social or communication deficits, not only will meeting new friends give him more opportunities to practice, but you'll be increasing the odds that he'll find a compatible friend or two.

Providing Opportunities for Social Experimentation

At every stage of social development, boys need to try out their fledgling skills. At first, providing opportunities at home (play dates, and the like) with family support may help make the process seem less intimidating. As your son becomes older and more socially adept, try expanding his arena of social experimentation.

■ *Facilitate group play.* If there are barriers to your son's finding a group of kids to play with (you live in a rural area, there are no kids his age in your development, and so on), make the extra effort to ensure that your son gets ample opportunities for socializing in different situations. Just as adults tend to have separate sets of friends— work colleagues, tennis partners, or old friends from college— children experience playing together differently depending on the venue: at school, on a team, informally in the yard. Notice which situations work best for your son.

■ *Support involvement in activities that expand his social circle.* An interscholastic league, a hobby that has a statewide convention, summer camp, or a visit to out-of-state relatives can all be good experiments about what happens with different places and people.

■ *Discuss group dynamics.* For boys with social challenges, preparation helps. Talk openly about what happens in groups and about how to adapt to groups at school versus those in his neighborhood or at your family's place of worship. Talk about peer pressure and discuss strategies for handling it.

Taking Chances

Without risk there can be no growth. At each stage of development, whether they're saying their first words or doing their first public speaking in school, boys need to stretch their abilities in the social realm. Sometimes, as adults, it's easy to forget how anxiety provoking it can be in achieving those milestones. Boys don't have the benefit of an adult perspective. They have a harder time saying, "Well, I'll give it my best try, and if I goof up, so what? Life goes on, and nobody will remember." The script going through your son's mind, as he considers his next social challenge, is more likely to sound like, "Oh no, I can't believe I have to do this. If I screw up, everyone will think I'm a loser, and I'll never live it down!" Just picking up the phone to make a call can make some boys break out in a sweat. (Suggest that he keep a list of "talking points" by the phone in case he "freezes.") Whatever the challenge, your job is to provide support. When boys fail to take chances, they lose the opportunity to grow and their self-esteem suffers.

■ *Encourage appropriate social risks.* Help your son stretch his social muscles by expanding his repertoire of abilities. You might coach your young son to approach new peers at the playground and introduce himself. For an older boy, you might suggest that he phone a friend who's mad at him. Help him stand up to a bully by role-playing and practicing verbal self-defense.

■ *Describe social failures as a normal and expected part of life.* "The first time I gave a speech I forgot some of my lines, too, but I got

■ ■ ■

Starting Over

After the loss of her husband, Leila's son Gary had gotten into a lot of trouble at his junior high school. It took a long time for Gary to work through his grief and rage. Unfortunately, he had aligned himself with the "bad" kids at school. He found it difficult to distance himself from them, and once he did, he found that the teachers and other kids still had him "pegged." Before he started high school, Leila took Gary to the school's guidance counselor, and he told her about his troubles. She assigned Gary to a homeroom that included many students Gary did not know and a teacher who was sympathetic to his problem. Slowly, he was able to rebuild a new network of friends and establish a fresh start. Could your son's reputation be limiting his social options? Does he need help in redefining who he is?

better at it." "I'm sorry Tracey turned you down. Obviously, she doesn't go for tall, handsome, smart boys."

■ *Help him rewrite the past.* If your son has developed a bad reputation or has hurt or alienated others through hostility, indifference, or confusion, let him know that the past doesn't have to define his future. Help him take the risk to redefine who he is and make amends when needed. If he needs a new set of friends, help him find some.

Being the Foundation

Providing a solid foundation of faith in your son's ability to succeed will help propel him through the turbulence of childhood and adolescence. Conversely, the doubts and criticisms of a parent can be devastating to a boy. Don't let frustration or anxiety obscure your message of conviction and belief in the potential of your child. Express your confidence in your son both verbally and through your actions.

■ *Be an unshakable foundation of belief in your son.* If your confidence in him wavers, seek support from someone who can restore your hope and help you move on. Our sons are works in progress and in most cases deserve the warmth and support of our enduring faith in what they can accomplish.

■ *Exercise care in how you speak about him to others.* Some parents let down their guard when discussing their son in front of family, friends, or even complete strangers. "I'm sorry, you have to ignore Albert; he can't help putting his foot in his mouth!" is not the kind thing your son should overhear. Don't assume that quiet boys aren't noticing you or that they're too young to understand.

Leadership

Helping your son develop leadership skills can be one of the most rewarding and fruitful things you do as a parent. A leader knows his own mind and can convey his thoughts and emotions in ways that motivate others to join with him. Raising a leader of good character can have exponentially positive effects on the future of individuals and communities—perhaps even whole nations.

When we talk about leaders, I don't necessarily mean a politician, a CEO, or even a particularly "powerful" person in the traditional sense. I do mean someone who knows who he is and what he stands for and who has the ability, courage, and common sense to live a life compatible with that identity and in positive relations with others. A boy can be articulate, kindhearted, and thoughtful, but if he can't take those skills and apply them through action when the situation requires, he hasn't been useful. Positive leadership is the ultimate application of good character.

■ *Emphasize the merits of social and emotional leadership.* Talk about great accomplishments that were achieved by gifted communicators and emotional leaders—Benjamin Franklin, Nelson Mandela, Gandhi, or one of my favorite examples, Antarctic maritime explorer Ernest Shackleton, who refused to leave his fellow explorers behind when disaster struck. See how their attributes are found among people in your own community.

■ *Invite your son's friends to be part of a group effort to make a social difference.* Whether it's a "race for a cure," a spring park cleanup, or a cause you champion yourselves, help your son expand his leadership skills in concert with his friends.

■ *Give your son the opportunity to make a positive difference.* You may have a relative who, as a child, contributed to the family by working during a time of special need. You may remember with pride an occasion when, at a young age, you took the initiative to help someone. Let your son have a chance to help the family in a time of crisis or reach out to the community with a bright idea.

■ *Express your pride in him.* When your son takes a leadership role and extends himself to others, be sure to let him know how proud you are. For most boys, it's nearly impossible to overstate how powerful a parent's approval is in shaping self-concept. When opportunity knocks, be generous with your approval.

Beyond Home

The dreams we have for our children form in the mists of our childhood. As good parents, we try to provide what we lacked, replicate what we valued, and reduce what we regretted or resented in our own youth. We can't avoid drawing from our childhood as a frame of reference for how we parent our sons, but we can distinguish between our own needs and those of our children while providing the basic moral guidance, support, and teaching they require. Each boy will require something a little different from his brother or friend, depending on his nature.

As if this complexity weren't engaging enough, we must also negotiate the world beyond home—the society we introduce our boys into. For most children, school is the first step they take toward moving independently in society. As parents, we know that school is, in part, a microcosm of the culture at large. School stretches the entire length of boyhood and most of adolescence. Your son's ability to feel a part of his school, and to negotiate the social challenges inherent in progressing from one grade to another, goes a long way toward shaping how he perceives himself. Yet just as your own childhood provides only an incomplete roadmap for parenting boys, your remembrances of school may have little to do with the social realities that your son encounters. What impact will school have on your son's communication and social development? Next, we'll consider ways you can practically work with school in your son's best interests.

TEN

Working with Schools

■ ■ ■

Most boys will attend school for at least twelve years following kindergarten. Twelve years of doing *anything* is a long time; because those twelve years occur during a period of intense personal development, from young child to young adult, their impact is enormous. School will likely serve as your son's introduction to, and his point of reference for, community life. In previous chapters we briefly touched on how school impacts your son's social development. Here we'll consider the opportunities and challenges of working with schools to foster your son's social and communication skills.

The School Environment

It's not unusual to find that boys who have been relatively well adjusted at home, and who may be comfortable playing with children who live nearby, face markedly greater challenges when it comes to school. It's easy to forget how different the school environment is from home or neighborhood; while school may provide an oasis of order, routine, and safety for some children, for most it represents a bit of a challenge, at least at first. One of the striking things about schools is how much energy flows through the hallways and the classrooms. It's easy for shy or withdrawn children to be overwhelmed. Depending on variables such as the environment and their own personalities, boys with angry or aggressive tendencies may benefit from the structure school provides and find their energies funneled into positive action. Conversely, they may find their worst impulses fueled by a desire to compete in a large arena, goaded by the compliance, or even encouragement, of their peers. Boys with learning disabilities can find the distractions and demands of a school environment especially hard to handle. The sheer number of students, and the volume and pace of activities, can be exciting, confusing, and sometimes daunting. Finding a sense of confidence and belonging in such a dynamic place is bound to be a hurdle for some boys. Boys of few words are particularly vulnerable to reacting to these challenges with stress, withdrawal, or confusion, because they have trouble accessing the primary pathways children use to understand and master the school environment—social communication skills.

Most peer interaction happens at school, and it occurs on a scale that is not usually replicated outside the classroom. School requires a great deal of socialization, including an acceptance of rules and an ability to understand the needs of a greater good. School is also where many children encounter their first experience of being judged by others; the objectivity of that judgment may be questioned, but acknowledgment of the *feeling* of being judged is rare. For some children, it will be the first time they are required to recognize that their individual needs will not always trump the needs of the group. They come to understand that they are one of many and that teachers will not favor them in the ways a parent might. When learning comes easily and school is fun, these facts may not create a significant emotional hurdle for a boy. However, when learning is more difficult and social ease at school doesn't come automatically, the environment can feel intimidating or hostile.

If you're concerned about your son's ability to cope with these social hurdles, do what you can to spend time at the school to get a sense of the environment so that you'll understand the social dynamics you might hear about from teachers or even from your son. Some of the "big picture" questions worth considering include:

- On the continuum from chaos to regimentation, what is the school's level or style of order?
- How does the school establish a sense of community? Are there many ways of "belonging"?
- In what ways does the school help children become "socialized" to the rules and expectations of the classroom?

Your consideration of these questions should be less focused on a search for the "right" answer than on an attempt to understand the personality of your son's school. Grasping how your son's school operates will help you coach him on how to be successful in that context. Remember that life is full of situations that require us to adapt; going to school is an important introduction to that reality.

One Size Does Not Fit All

Children thrive in different size groups. While some children may do exceptionally well in small groups or one-on-one, other children do best in larger groups. The focused attention of small groups may make some boys feel self-conscious about communicating. When they feel the spotlight is on them too strongly, they will often withdraw or adopt a form of camouflage for protection. Yet a teacher who notices the special needs of a self-conscious boy may be able to successfully integrate him into the group and also use the close attention to draw out his self-expression. A large classroom or school may offer too many distractions to encourage social and communication focus. But some boys enjoy the diversity, resources, and high energy level of a large school. A large school may also provide more potential niches where your son can find success.

Larger groups can cause boys to feel lost in a crowd and therefore anxious. Suddenly having a lot of competition can bring out the

■ ■ ■

Understanding your son's temperament and which environments he enjoys can help you predict or understand which school situations will encourage his development. Does your young son charge into a large birthday party with a smile on his face or need encouragement to join the group? Once he's there, does he join in the party games well, or do you have trouble with misbehavior because he's so excited? Would your teen prefer an outdoor jam with twenty friends or hiking with a buddy or two? Consider his experiences with day care, religious education, or recreational activities that involve being with other kids. Does he like small group activities or getting into the mix with the whole group? Take special note if his mood or level of performance varies in small or large groups. What have you and his instructors observed?

worst in boys who are assertive and used to ruling the roost, either at home or in their neighborhoods. Some retreat in a sulk, while others increase their assertiveness to the point of aggression in an effort to be noticed. Shy or withdrawn boys may give up without even trying or may develop unhealthy ways of dealing with the stress of the situation. Toby, eleven, had transitioned from a small parochial school to a larger public school when his parents moved. "He was always somewhat involved in school," said his father, "and the sisters did a good job in bringing him out. But after he transferred, his grades took a nosedive. When we spoke with his teacher, she said Toby just looks off into the distance and kind of disappears. After a lot of prodding and guesswork, we figured out that he had built up a fantasy about being an alien who had to blend in. I think he had no idea how to cope, so he just shut down and withdrew into this make-believe universe where he could imagine himself as important and special." Toby's parents were able to move him back to a smaller school the next year. "We balanced the risks of another transition against the benefits of a small class size. The school he was at was excellent, and we really liked his teacher, but it wasn't a good fit for Toby."

Try to gauge your son's social comfort in different-size groups before he begins school. Parent–teacher conferences are generally held partway through the school year, so you may decide to talk to your son's teacher before the school year commences if you have concerns. Deanna, mother of six-year-old Harding, took this approach. "I let his new teacher know that he tends to be shy at first and that we've found the more you encourage him to join in, the more stubborn and withdrawn he gets. He's a little nervous in new situations and resents it when you put the focus on him. At home we've found that if we ignore him a little, he sort of softens up, and we just casually bring him into the conversation, almost like we didn't notice that he came over. He's kind of like a cat who won't sit in your lap if you invite him, but if you ignore him, he's there. I actually explained it this way to his teacher, and she smiled and nodded, so I think she gets it about boys like Harding."

Teachers as Collaborators

While we rely on our own observations and judgments to help boys live up to their social potential, let's not underestimate the ability of teachers to be our collaborators in this process. While no one probably knows your son like you do, his teacher is watching him in a situation that you rarely have an opportunity to observe (the classroom) and has the benefit of a different relationship with him. So with a second set of eyes, any hypothesis you might have about his nature or ability can be tested. Brent, age nine, was, according to his parents, "a holy terror"—defiant, destructive, and impertinent. Yet he did well in school and seemed to mention his teacher a lot. His mother said, "I couldn't wait until we had our parent–teacher conference. I asked his teacher, 'Does he behave for you? What are you doing?' and he said that Brent was very bright, liked to be in charge, and needed to have a job." It turned out that Brent's teacher had assigned him the task of being a class moderator, helping to resolve disputes that emerged among other children. "We realized that Brent didn't have a lot of opportunities for leadership or responsibility in our home, but when we started to put him to work, he was happier and more cooperative. It just never occurred to me that he wanted a job!" Schools provide a wealth of information and talent when it comes to helping boys become effective social communicators. The feedback available to parents through school can save months, if not years, of time in coming to understand the challenges of an individual child.

■ ■ ■

If you have a young son . . . Ask his teacher which children he gets along with best and invite them to your house or take them along on an outing. Observing them together will give you a chance to find out whom your son feels emotionally safe with and what traits he responds to in others. You may have to be more circumspect with your teenage son, but if you occasionally drive him and his friends and make your home "teen friendly," with a space to congregate, snacks, and a music system, you should be able to make similar observations.

One of the great benefits of the school community is that it does offer a place for your son to attain a degree of status and achievement beyond academics. George Bartlett, headmaster of the South Kent School in Connecticut from 1969 to 1989, often asked his students to be involved in the upkeep of the campus. Doing such useful work "made them important to the community and helped build their sense of who they were." Chuck Canfield, a special education teacher for fifteen years and fourth-grade teacher for ten years in the Allentown, Pennsylvania, school system, says, "Sometimes I put [his fourth-grade] kids in important positions, such as monitoring attendance or carrying messages . . . there are many ways they can feel important." Boys relish action and leadership, and experienced teachers provide opportunities for both.

The Right Teacher

One year of school may be very different from the next. Many times I've met with parents convinced of their son's "lack of ability," only to find out the next year that having the right teacher—one who is a good fit for his needs—proves a suspected diagnosis was wrong. While even the best teacher cannot be all things to all children, a good teacher can bring out the best in most children. Teachers who bring passion, commitment, and insight to their work are our national treasures. (If our society is to promote diverse role models, we need a public forum to acknowledge the talent and accomplishments of teachers and allied professionals to counterbalance the emphasis we place on sports and entertainment. Like it or not, our sons will be attracted to the role models our society celebrates most.) When your son is fortunate enough to have such a teacher, enjoy the opportunity to collaborate with him or her to bring out the best in your son. George Bartlett talked about searching for teachers who could do this. "It's not just that people have to love kids—they all love their own—they have to love *other* people's kids." Will all your son's teachers have that capability? Probably not, yet within every school there are teachers who have the wisdom and empathy to give a positive shape to your son's social development. Actively participate in his education, talk with other parents, and visit the school. You'll find out which teachers stand out and maximize your chances of finding those who will be a good fit for your son. Dr. Sue Straeter, assistant director of Hillside School, a private school for children with learning disabilities in eastern Pennsylvania, said that effective parents "have to be involved in conferences, observe their children in class, ask good questions, and read the 'homebook' [notes from a child's teacher sent home each day]."

This is especially true if your son has significant learning challenges or related neurodevelopmental problems. When your son is

■ ■ ■

Love the One You're With

If your son's teacher is not a good fit for him, but circumstances prevent you from moving him from the class, it's time to get creative.

- Try, try, try to form a positive alliance with the teacher. Even if you don't agree with his approach, or if she doesn't "click" with your son, keep the lines of communication open.
- Enlist the support of other school personnel, such as guidance counselors, aides, coaches, or the principal. If they're aware of your son's challenges, they can do a lot to mitigate a less-than-perfect classroom experience.
- Be a partner with your son. Appropriately acknowledge the limitations of his current situation and let him know you're concerned and supportive. "I know Mrs. Smith is unusually strict, but let's think of some new ideas about how to get along with her," or "I'm sorry that Mr. Jones ignores you. Although I don't want you to misbehave to get his attention, I want you to keep raising your hand. And I want you to remember what the class was about, so we can talk about it when you come home. You'll have a lot to teach me!"

starting at a disadvantage, it's even more important to be selective about his teachers. Don't assume every teacher will have the appropriate training, motivation, or resources to help your son work through his difficulties. Edward, father of a sixth-grade boy whose grades had plummeted, had met with his son's teacher. "Ed Jr. has been diagnosed with some learning disabilities, but they're mild enough so that he can be in a regular classroom. He gets reading support three times a week outside class. His teacher is a good guy, has been there for years, everyone likes him. But he has a notion that kids with special learning problems just need extra effort and a good attitude to keep up. He kept telling Eddie things like 'If you put your mind to it, you could do better' or 'Even though it's not fun, sometimes we have to work hard.' I agree with those statements in general, but Eddie felt embarrassed and frustrated when he kept on saying them. Eddie was trying, but he felt that his efforts weren't being respected, so he stopped trying as hard. We eventually decided he might do better with a different teacher and asked the school to change his classroom. She's not quite as experienced, but seems much better at working with him. We're pleased with the change in his attitude."

Parent–Teacher Conferences

Whatever the purpose of the conference—from pre-school-year consultation to regularly scheduled meetings to requested conferences—it pays to be strategic when preparing for a conference with your son's teacher. The time your son's teacher can spend with you will likely be limited, and you don't want to find yourself wishing you had remembered to ask about important concerns after the fact. Make notes about the questions you want to ask, whether they're about how this teacher observes your son, classroom protocol, or the school's philosophy, programs, and special education services.

One question you might begin with is, "What are my son's specific strengths?" Astute teachers will have something positive to say about your child. In fact, the best will start with this without being asked. It could be a pleasant surprise to you, or it could confirm your own observation. Generally, this will provide a springboard for further discussion about strategies for capitalizing on those strengths. It will also make any subsequent negative feedback easier for your son's teacher to deliver (remember, no one likes to be the bearer of bad news!) and for you to hear. Even if you disagree with the information you receive, it's important for you to have. Asking about strengths will also help you get a sense of the teacher's general disposition toward your son. If she or he struggles to find a specific strength, consider the options. Is your son so withdrawn in the class that his teacher doesn't know him well? Is your son behaving badly? Does his teacher lack experience or have an uninformed perspective of the behavior of boys? (Keep an open mind—you're just warming up, and sometimes a person who connects beautifully with a classroom full of children is not as eloquent with their parents.)

Also, take good notes about what your son's teacher tells you. If you have concerns or need further clarification, don't hesitate to follow up with either your son's teacher or administrative personnel as required. The important thing is to come away with some meeting of the minds about your son's needs and how to meet them. Leslie, whose son Christopher is in third grade, had met with his teacher to discuss some minor disciplinary problems. "Chris can be tough. Academically he can just about keep up, but socially he's immature. He has a hard time articulating when he needs some clarification or is feeling frustrated and tends to act out rather than ask for help. Last year he had a fantastic teacher. He had a way of dealing with him that was almost like a man-to-man discussion. He'd set out his expectations, say 'I know you can handle this job if you do it step by step it, so just let me know when you're ready for the next part,' and Chris knocked himself out to please him. This year his teacher is new. She's trying hard to establish authority in the class and has set a lot of new rules. When he loses track during a project and starts wandering or chatting, she disciplines, rather than prompts, him. While she feels she's being attentive and setting high standards, Chris thinks she's picking on him. He doesn't see that she's being hard on him because she wants him to succeed. Until we met, she didn't realize how Chris was responding emotionally. I give her credit, though—she has agreed to give him a trial period of working more collaboratively with her, if he can demonstrate more responsible behavior in the classroom."

A teacher who has a positive attitude and conveys his or her belief in your child is a tremendous ally. Overall, just like good parenting, the classroom paradigm should be based more on rewards than punishment. The trend in many schools is to have students sign contracts (often effective) or track their behavior with a chart. Charts and visual aids can be particularly helpful for boys with impulsivity or executive control problems, because they provide a visual prompt for positive behavior. Charts can be highly individualized—one boy's goal could be "acknowledge and greet classmates each day," while another's could be "raise hand to answer at least three questions each day." Describing his teaching philosophy, George Bartlett said, "A lot of teachers start at 100 and subtract. I start at 0 and add—that's the way parents should think about their kids. Issuing ultimatums doesn't work. You have to show kids you respect them. [When kids are doing well] somebody has to notice, and somebody has to *show* that they notice." I emphatically agree with this perspective. As a corollary, when I work with schools to implement behavioral modification, I emphasize that we should spend much more time rewarding boys for what they do well than punishing them for what they do wrong. Unfortunately, with the best of intentions, some teachers undermine their own efforts by establishing a system where a child starts the day with *X* number of points and then has them taken away with each behavioral infraction. *This is not an effective approach to teaching positive behavior.* Instead, we should be stimulating creativity and encouraging thought to be focused on how to earn points. Then you're setting the paradigm for mastery and achievement and the positive psychological rewards that motivate boys. Boys are much less engaged by figuring out how to protect what they already have than by the idea of earning more acknowledgment. Aren't you more motivated to work for a pay increase than for maintaining your current salary?

When you think your son isn't being understood adequately, or when you perceive a real philosophical disconnect between you and your son's teacher, it's time to consider alternative options. If your son is seeing a psychologist or a speech–language therapist, don't hesitate to ask if he or she can be included in school conferences when it's in your son's best interest. It's often advantageous to have multiple people at the table brainstorming when there are problems to be solved. One reason is that the *conceptualization* of what's happening for your son will have an awful lot to do with the type of intervention provided. It's important to have the greatest insight at the point where conceptualizing the problem is taking place. Sometimes interventions are developed around an *assumption* about a boy. Make sure you and your son's teachers have a sound concept and good level of agreement about what's happening with your son before taking action. After all, if you misdiagnose the issue, your interventions are bound to fail!

During a teleconference at the beginning of the school year, I was speaking with several teachers, a guidance counselor, the school principal, and the parents of eleven-year-old Russell about how to help him socially in his new school. His difficulty in getting along with peers had resulted in escalating incidents of disruptive behavior. Russell had confided to me that he felt "despised" by other kids but could not explain why they would feel this way toward him. He told me, "I'm not going to let them get away with it anymore. I don't care what happens." He had spent part of the previous year at his new school and immediately had problems fitting in. Russell and his parents assumed that with the start of a new school year he would be more easily assimilated into the flow of school life. But during our conference some interesting observations emerged. One teacher noted that Russell rarely made any type of positive attempt to inter- act with other students. She remarked that the problem wasn't so much that other students didn't like him but that they just didn't know what to make of him. She explained that Russell's comments were frequently "off task." While he had an excellent vocabulary, he often talked above his peers, in effect alienating them. Hearing this teacher's insights, others in the meeting realized they saw a similar social phenomenon in Russell's peer interactions. Consequently, our discussion shifted to focusing on how to teach Russell the verbal skills needed to be accepted by other students and how to prompt him to practice these skills on a regular basis.

When interventions are to be applied in school, one of the most effective strategies is to plan a follow-up meeting at the end of the first meeting to establish accountability. In a busy school, the best in- tentions can get "lost in the wash" because new situations are arising every day!

The Right School

If you have a choice about which school your son will attend, you'll undoubtedly be looking at a variety of factors: academic rigor, extra- curricular opportunities, expense, commute, class size, teaching prac- tice and philosophy, to name a few. Don't forget to consider how these factors will influence his communication skills and social devel- opment. Marybeth and Tom sent both of their sons to Tom's alma mater, a military academy. They thought their elder son's aggression would be channeled more positively in a highly structured environ- ment, but it was their shy younger son who benefited, becoming much more articulate and confident. Their older son eventually found a better fit at a small, coed Quaker school, where collaboration was strongly emphasized over competition.

We've already talked about how the size of the classroom and school can influence your son's development. Some other points to consider include:

■ *All boys or coed?* While fewer single-sex schools exist today, those that remain are generally highly experienced in motivating and teaching boys. Some parents find their sons enjoy being considered the focus, rather than the potential disruption, of the classroom!

Boys who are extremely self-conscious or distracted around girls can benefit from an opportunity to devote attention to academics and find this success mirrored in their social and communication skills. Conversely, some parents feel their sons are equally or better served in a coed environment that reflects the world they will know post-graduation.

■ *Social support.* Does the school have an environment and policies that support boys' healthy social communication skills? Are there antibullying, peer mentoring, dispute resolution programs?

■ *A place to shine.* Some schools develop a reputation for excellence in one area at the expense of others. If a school is known for its Ivy League acceptance rate or undefeated football team, are there opportunities and resources for boys if they strive for different accomplishments?

■ *Expressive communication and language arts.* Does the school place high value on developing excellent communication skills? Are reading and language arts emphasized? Are student achievement levels in these areas acceptable? Are the school newspaper, yearbook, drama program, and student government well supported?

These questions can likely be answered by meeting with the school's admissions office, administrators, guidance counselors, or teachers. If your son is at a public school, please get actively involved in its parent–teacher association. Take the time to meet with your son's teachers and understand their teaching philosophy, including their thoughts on your son's specific challenges. Schools that will not accommodate your reasonable requests for information—no matter how "exclusive"—should raise a red flag. Parents need more than generalized answers to be effective collaborators in their sons' education.

> ■ ■ ■
> Research indicates that one of the best predictors of a boy's academic success is his *father's* participation in his school's parent–teacher organization.

Special Education for Social Learning

Among the many school options parents have—private, public, charter, and parochial—the type that may be least familiar to parents are those that meet the needs of children with specific learning problems. Special education is not limited to developmentally disabled children; there are, for example, schools for highly gifted students who happen to have learning disabilities. If you feel your son is having trouble adapting to his school, please consider other available options within your area and budget. (We often assume that the "sticker price" of a private education will be our out-of-pocket cost; it's worth investigating loans and scholarships for education at the elementary or secondary level if it makes the difference in your son's ability to achieve a quality education.) The Internet offers a wealth of information about schools in virtually every area of the country; you can also find directories at your local library. Private academic advisers are also available, although their services come at a price, of course. Most private schools will welcome you to take a tour of their facilities and will make an appointment for you to meet with staff to discuss what curricula they follow and how they work to meet the needs of children with social learning challenges.

Getting the Assessment Your Son Needs If He Has a Learning Disability

Assessment is a broad term that can have different meanings to different people. It can cover anything from an observational assessment made by an experienced teacher to a formal evaluation done by a pediatric neuropsychologist specializing in learning disabilities. Regardless of what level of assessment takes place, it's important that some type of evaluation occur. This process marks the beginning of your attempts to be more analytical about your son's needs and also sets in motion the process by which any interventions deemed necessary will be offered. Sue Straeter believes that learning disability assessments often point to specific social liabilities that can help a school get a jump start on a child's special needs. She notes that using the results of assessment, private therapeutic schools can make suggestions to parents that teachers in a public school may hesitate to make.

Virtually all schools have some type of professional person who completes formal assessments of children with learning disabilities and/or emotional adjustment difficulties. Usually they are school psychologists, who have great expertise in testing a child's ability and achievement and may offer additional insight about behavioral problems, especially ADHD, that interfere with learning. Parents of children in public schools have a right to request an evaluation for specialized educational intervention. This type of intervention is called an *individualized education plan*, or IEP. An IEP identifies specific objectives that your son's school team will address for remediation. In addition, the school identifies how it will measure its progress in meeting these goals and typically sets a schedule for assessing such progress. Because an IEP is a highly formalized approach to intervention, it has some substantial advantages. Parents often appreciate an IEP because they know they will be getting regular feedback from schools about the progress of their children. Schools are sometimes hesitant to identify a student as requiring an IEP because children change so much from year to year and even within a single school year. A school's first instinct may be to take a "wait and see" attitude, making small modifications it hopes will resolve a problem. An unfortunate reality is that some schools also hesitate to initiate an IEP because it means additional work for teachers and related school personnel, and they may simply lack the resources. Teachers have become accustomed to having many children with IEPs in the classroom. Although it's certainly ideal to provide each child with the optimal education for his or her specific liabilities, you can imagine how difficult it must be to teach thirty students, half of whom may have some type of identified special educational need. How can a teacher practically keep track of all those needs on a daily basis?

In addition, children today are arguably less prepared to attend to classroom business. In discussing the changes he's seen in students over the past twenty-six years, and how he goes about keeping his classroom interesting, educator Chuck Canfield says, "We're competing with GameBoys. Their attention spans are shorter—they are more difficult to engage . . . I have to be an actor!" Teachers who can meet these challenges—juggling the diverse needs of students while captivating an increasingly overstimulated and inattentive group of students—are the unsung heroes of our time. We rarely recognize the extraordinary talent required of teachers who perform this very valuable service and who stand tough in the face of complex and mounting neurodevelopmental challenges among children, especially boys.

As we discussed in Chapter 7, social learning disabilities are sometimes overlooked relative to more specific learning disabilities involving reading or math skills. However, social learning disabilities present lifelong deficits that impair a boy's ability to achieve his potential in adulthood. Intervention can be difficult but is critical. Sue Straeter agrees: "learning problems require a lifetime of learning by parents . . . helping children is hard work."

Nonverbal learning disabilities and social learning problems can have a pronounced impact on boys' development. If your son has such a problem, please don't hesitate to assert his needs with his school, including a request for a detailed plan to bolster these aspects of his social self-development. He may require several sessions per week with a speech–language therapist who can assist with pragmatic communication, or he may need to see a reading specialist to enhance his enjoyment of written material and consequently improve his understanding of expressive language. The earlier children can be identified as needing intervention, the better.

On my way back to the airport in Atlanta, after having given a talk about the social development of boys at a recent conference, I struck up a conversation with a cab driver who was curious about the details of my talk. He listened quite carefully and then divulged his own story: "When I was in school, no one heard of disabilities like they talk about today. But when I got out of school, I figured out something was wrong. I never learned all the things I was supposed to. Driving a cab, I've listened to a lot of people, and I guess I finally figured out what people are trying to say, if you know what I mean. I kind of know what language they're talking, and it's made a big difference." We owe our sons our careful attention and, when necessary, our advocacy to see that they get the help they need early in their schooling. As hard as it is to discover that you have a learning disability, it's tragic to find out long after the optimal window for intervention has closed.

There will be times when your son's school, despite all best efforts, is not able to provide the detailed kind of assessment he may need. If this occurs, it will be important to find a psychologist who can do the required testing. This will involve looking at language skills, social perceptual skills, and any related learning problems your son has. We'll examine what's involved in such an evaluation in the next chapter. For now, consider an assessment a roadmap—to provide direction about where you're going, what should be happening along the way, and where you will eventually arrive.

Because educational systems vary so much, you'll have to spend some time researching how to go about getting special accommodations from schools. Your board of education, parent–teacher organization, or state learning disabilities association should be able to give you an idea about where to start.

Building Success in the Classroom

Boys have all different types of communication challenges, and even those problems that have been diagnosed will be expressed differently, reflecting the uniqueness of your son's mind and personality. Consider two boys assessed as having "pragmatic communication deficits": One consistently misreads the intentions of others and as a result misinterprets the feelings and thoughts that his peers have about him, often unnecessarily feeling disliked. Another makes similar attribution errors yet is more aggressive by nature and expresses his confusion through hostility or socially disruptive behavior. Although the diagnostic labels could be identical, the interventions for these boys would be significantly different. It's important to be adaptable and to apply team creativity and collaboration wherever possible. Within that flexibility, I've found five basic strategies useful in coaching boys to improve social communication:

1. When a boy has a social communication problem, sometimes we forget to discuss the issue with the most important person—the boy himself. Explain clearly and in appropriate detail what your expectations are: "I want you to look me in the eye and answer my questions with friendly words," or "I would like to help you be able to tell me what's bothering you before you storm off." Until you've clearly communicated your expectations, you haven't given a boy the best chance of winning your approval.

2. Whenever possible, provide some type of visual learning reference that helps a boy understand what is expected of him. A favorite intervention of mine is to ask schools to videotape a child when he's having an exceptionally good day so that he knows exactly what "good" means. A boy who sees himself talking and interacting successfully with peers is imprinted with a specific idea of how to act at the future prompting of his teacher. (Although this type of intervention requires some extra effort with logistics, it may ultimately be the most expe-

ditious route to teaching some social skills—a picture can be worth a thousand words).

3. Ask teachers/aides to provide consistent coaching throughout the school day. This means taking the time to remind a boy about the social dimension of what's taking place, what type of transition will be occurring, and what specific challenges he'll face within the next thirty to sixty minutes. "Keenan, your group will be voting on who presents your project to the class. If they pick you, will you agree to try?" "Why don't you pick Chandler for your partner, since you forgot him last time?"

4. Be as positive as you possibly can in reinforcing successful communication when it occurs. When you receive a favorable report from school, let your son know his teacher has noticed he's done something well. Boys love to feel proud of their accomplishments and acknowledged for something worthy of adult approval. Make sure you unambiguously state your approval and combine that with other forms of loving acknowledgment, such as a pat on the back or a hug when appropriate.

5. If your son has had a problem and the intervention plan you've designed in cooperation with your son's school is not working, change it! Don't wait a year of your son's life to determine whether a plan is going to be successful. I'm not suggesting that you give up if change is slow—substantive change is usually gradual, and you can expect ups and downs. But if the overall trend is not positive, or if there's no indication of change within several weeks, a better plan or a different approach is usually required.

Some of the following school-based, specific interventions may be helpful to your son, depending on the nature of his communication deficits. You might want to talk to his teacher about the possibility of initiating some of these strategies:

■ *Facilitating social groups within the classroom.* Some schools have programs to help kids interact with each other, resolve conflicts, or buddy up.

■ *Providing social narration for boys while they are watching educational media or interacting with peers on the playground.* Teachers sometimes use videos or computer programs specifically designed to build social communication skills, while others capitalize on situations as they occur in the classroom to bring up points about interacting with peers and communicating with others.

■ *Providing careful supervision of play at recess and other times when boys are casually interacting with peers.* Sadly, fewer schools now offer recess, as liability issues and performance mandates increase. However, providing children with time to "blow off steam" and meet informally has substantial social benefits. However, unsupervised recess, lunch, or hallway travel is prime time for social exchanges that can be especially deleterious to boys of few words, who are often victims or perpetrators of teasing and bullying.

■ *Modeling appropriate communication skills, including rephrasing when necessary within the course of the class.* Some schools suggest scripts for conflict resolution, asking permission, and sharing.

■ *Providing a child with preferential seating toward the front of the class so that he's more responsive to what the teacher is saying and so that he has an easier opportunity to express himself.*

■ *Providing a peer mentor to assist with various types of social skills, such as introductions, getting to know new friends, or conflict resolution.*

Moving from One Grade to the Next

One of the most remarkable things about boys with apparent learning or social problems is how the complexion of those problems can change from year to year. As boys' peer groups change, as their teachers change, and as they grow older, sometimes a behavior that was a problem only six months earlier resolves itself, while yet new problems emerge. For this reason it's helpful to understand these problems within a developmental context. Average development implies the convergence of a spectrum of traits within broad parameters; the required balancing act is to decide whether a boy will outgrow something (no action needed) or be exponentially harmed by inaction. We sometimes rush to identify the specific syndrome or "disorder" that labels a child's behavior. While this may have advantages, insofar as a label is often required to receive school or state-mandated services, it can also prematurely foreclose our psychological understanding of a child. Further, such labels sometimes stigmatize boys in a way that the teacher in the next grade has a relatively low expectation for his potential performance. One teacher has confided to me that he has decided not to review the evaluation reports provided to teachers at the beginning of the school year before he meets and gets to know these children. While he doesn't want to ignore important information about his students, he doesn't want to be influenced by the reports to have low expectations for his students' ability to achieve.

A famous psychological experiment undertaken in the 1960s, led by Dr. Robert Rosenthal, involved a group of elementary school teachers in San Francisco. They were told that students on a particular list could expected to be academically high achieving as determined by psychological testing and that they should have high expectations for their performance. In reality, these students had been selected randomly. The experiment revealed that these children did in fact do well, not because of higher levels of ability, but because their teachers expected them to. This phenomenon is called the "Rosenthal effect," and it continues to resonate with psychologists and educators because it shows us that our beliefs about people shape how we interact with them on multiple levels. The study also demonstrated that children can detect our perceptions and will respond accordingly.

What if you told your son's teacher, "I want to give you a heads-up because he's been diagnosed with ADHD, but I'd like you to observe him and then to meet with you to get your own impression of his capabilities before we get into what his evaluation says." Now imagine if you forwarded your son's psychological report to the teacher before she met your son and asked to meet with her before the class started to discuss classroom interventions. While both approaches might be appropriate in different circumstances, and although you want to make your son's teacher aware of any learning challenges he may have, it's worth considering how the timing and context in which you communicate this information will influence his teacher's opinion.

Focusing on Peer Interaction

One of the most useful windows into your son's social development is to watch his interaction with peers. In fact, school may be the ideal place to assess interpersonal skills. Although most parents cannot be casually present at school, by volunteering to be an assistant in your son's classroom, helping a teacher's aide, or simply attending school activities you can learn about what occurs socially for your son on a daily basis. One parent said, "I was helping with a school raffle. One of the other parents was making signs and asked, 'How do you spell lacrosse?' Immediately, two kids turned toward my son. They said, 'Conrad can tell you! He can spell anything!' I've always been worried that other kids didn't notice him, but it showed me that his classmates had some admiration for him and could be friendly if he gave them the chance. I don't think Conrad would have ever told me that, even if he had realized it. But seeing the kids appreciate him gave us something to work with."

Because boys are receiving feedback and forming their self-concept on a cumulative basis, teachers and parents can be helpful by observing how peers react to them. Sometimes boys don't realize the signals they're sending to other people and as a result don't necessarily understand or feel responsible for the type of reaction they get from others. Nonetheless, boys *are* receiving feedback daily. By watching how others react to them, we can gain some insight into how boys feel about themselves and how they're constructing their social world.

Listening closely to the kind of language boys use on the playground, for example, is very useful. Does your son know how to talk to peers differently than he would to an adult? Does he know how to relate to both boys and girls in productive ways? There are few things more frustrating to a child than feeling as though he is shut out of a social group. When this happens, teachers and parents can teach boys how to "break into" social groups or facilitate social interaction that makes it easier for them to become involved. Naturally, this is easier at schools where some latitude is given to teachers or at schools that are in a position to support such experiential learning. Chuck Canfield said, "We used to have a twenty-minute meeting each day, learning to give and accept compliments, sharing, and introducing. It was a way to make all types of kids part of a group. Because of time constraints, we can't do these things anymore." During the many conversations I've had with public school teachers, they've echoed this concern. At a time when children's need for social connection is greater than ever, there seems to be less and less time for teaching those skills and nurturing that connection. Parents can help compensate by providing opportunities for group socialization and teaching these skills at home.

Beware of Bullies

Perhaps the most detrimental type of peer interaction a boy can face is to be confronted by a bully. Because of their communicative or social deficits, some boys are, unfortunately, easy targets for other boys, who can make them feel even less powerful and more socially anxious. Sadly, all schools have bullies, although how schools deal with the issue varies tremendously. Bullies come in many shapes and sizes; some are extroverted and aggressive, while others tend to be more subtle and coercive. In whatever shape bullies may appear, they inhibit the social development of other children. Through an intimidating presence, bullies make it more difficult for children to experiment with social communication. Bullies heighten a boy's sense of anxiety by making his fear of failure more pronounced. When your son tells you he's being teased or bullied by someone, take him seriously. Sometimes we hesitate to take action because we don't know what to do or we fear making matters worse. Other times we minimize the pain and trauma bullying can inflict. Make an effort to investigate the situation with school personnel. If you're told your son is exaggerating, ask him for more specific facts or see if you or your representative (and you can be inventive here—a trusted school buddy or sibling can be your proxy) can be present during the part of the day when he complains he is being harassed. *Under no circumstances should you continue to allow your son to attend a school where he is being bullied on a daily basis.* Although schools can be overcrowded and professional staff may be overwhelmed, there is *no* excuse for allowing a child to be subjected to daily taunts or bullying. The verbal assaults alone can be unbelievably ugly and have lifelong repercussions.

As parents, our gut reaction may be to teach our sons to stand up to bullies. When our sons are in pain, we experience it vicariously, and the situation can make us very angry. We might suggest what they should "say back" to bullies or, as is the case with some fathers, fantasize that our sons will physically teach a bully a lesson. With the best of intentions, we can end up burdening our sons with an obligation to defend our own pride!

Some parents will sign up their kids for martial arts courses or teach their sons how to "street fight." Although these instincts may be natural and human, they are rarely effective solutions to a bully problem. While we can coach our sons on the art of verbal self-defense and help them develop the inner strength and confidence that tends to ward off bullies, these are interventions that take time. Bullies who use the threat of force are often intimidating because they are big, strong, and can't be easily vanquished. Children who hurt with words attack those who are unwilling or unable to respond to such assaults. In the curious social world of school, sometimes what an adult would consider to be an effective verbal defense doesn't help, while a juvenile taunt takes off like wildfire and becomes understood by the kids as a devastating put-down. One young boy could not bear to go to school because he was being called a "turtle," but the taunt was used to indicate his position as a social outcast, rather than a comment on his speed or appearance.

Often we forget that our sons are being bullied precisely because they are physically or expressively vulnerable; an intense flurry of indignant coaching can backfire. In fact, what happens for most boys is that they feel even greater pressure to live up to parental expectations and as a result shut down, telling you less and less about what is actually happening. That's if you find out at all—it simply doesn't occur to many boys to let their parents know about teasing at school. Remember, boys prefer a sense of mastery, and when they are humiliated, confused, or frightened, they stop talking. You may see the glum expression and daily depression, but no longer get specific information as to what is leading to that disposition.

So what is a parent to do? You must react, but your interventions are unlikely to succeed quickly and could further alienate your son. Certainly, if your son is being teased or bullied, you should help him build the preventive and defensive skills (self-confidence, good social pragmatics, verbal dexterity, and so forth) that help ward off attacks. Although you may wish to contact the parents of the bully directly, this is often ill advised, and, unfortunately, potentially dangerous, if you don't already know them. This is a situation, however, where it can be practical to look to your son's teacher or school to intercede. The good news is that schools are increasingly aware of the dangers of bullying, and many have programs in place to address the issue. Some teachers keep a book where kids can anonymously write about being teased or bullied, and classroom meetings are held every week. Chuck Canfield keeps such a book and says it's important to teach children to make "I" rather than "You" statements (for example, "I'm angry" rather than "You make me angry") and for teachers to assign real consequences for teasing and bullying.

Claudette, whose seventh-grade son was being constantly taunted for his small stature, said, "Luke was being teased, and he tried ignoring it and using humor to defuse it, but nothing worked. I asked him if he wanted me to go to the school, but he was adamant that he didn't want me to do that. So I agreed not to, but asked him to find one teacher he thought he could trust and ask his advice. So he mentioned it to his gym teacher, because a lot of the ridicule happened in the locker room. Luke was low key about the whole thing, but he casually let me know that the next time those boys started in on him the gym teacher was all over it; he apparently let these kids know that he considered their insults to Luke to be insults to him; he said they were disrespecting themselves and, as he put it, 'my gym.' Because the boys respect his authority, it carried a lot of weight, and the incident went all over the school. It's been much better for Luke ever since. I owe his gym teacher big time!"

Teasing and bullying are often systemic, and like most cancers, are best dealt with early on, by the top school administration, with a zero tolerance policy. Every child has a right to receive an education without fear of physical or emotional abuse; we wouldn't put up with it at home or in the workplace, and it has no place in our schools.

What If Your Son Is the Bully?

Interestingly, boys of few words are likely to be both the victims and the perpetrators of bullying behavior. As we have seen, some of these boys are prone to angry and aggressive behavior. Boys whose frustration or aggression vents itself on classmates are not unusual. This type of bullying may reflect expressive language deficits and an inability to be assertive in a socially constructive way. Please don't feel resistant to hearing information from teachers if they report that your son is teasing or bullying others. Instead of drawing conclusions that this means your son has an antisocial personality or conduct problem (if you don't really believe such a thing is true), investigate what kinds of triggers are causing your son's behavior. Sometimes there's a "ringleader" who is spurring the other boys on, and they participate because they're afraid of becoming his next victim. A teacher may see your son responding to an insult or attack without having witnessed the precipitating event. Yet be thorough in your investigation and willing to accept the word of eyewitnesses. If it turns out that your son is picking on another child, talk to him frankly about your desire to see him act in more positive social ways and assign serious consequences for noncompliance.

It may be especially important for fathers to model how their sons can be both strong leaders and kind people and to express disappointment in their sons when they become aggressive or use bullying-type tactics to assert their dominance within a peer group. Disappointment is a very powerful motivator for boys. It's okay to express to a child that you feel disappointed in his behavior. If your child has a good and healthy relationship with you, he will not see this as an end to that relationship or as an insurmountable hurdle. Rather, he's more likely to understand that you care about the behavioral choices that he makes and consequently attempt to change his behavior in a way that is consistent with your own ideals.

Ignoring the issue in the hope that it will go away is tantamount to approval and, as one father found out, potentially expensive. He learned that his son had been verbally harrassing another boy when the boy's mother called to complain. Thinking this mother was overreacting, and resentful of her accusations, he did nothing. To his astonishment, he found himself being sued along with the school district. Although the suit was eventually dismissed, he spent a considerable sum on legal fees and was required to pay the costs of court-mandated evaluation and counseling for his son. Although he might have averted this scenario, arguably, it was money well spent!

Boys who feel academically unsuccessful, who are impulsive or have difficulty "reading" others, and boys who lack empathy or the expressive skills to manage their emotions, are all at risk of becoming bullies. Just as we wish to protect our sons from being bullied, we should wish to keep them safe from becoming bullies, an experience equally detrimental to a boy's emotional development. Bullying is a perverse path to feelings of mastery and competence, grinding the healthy development of character and growth of empathy to a halt. Parents are on the front line of defense in this effort; and in this case the best defense is a strong offense. Let your son know that cruelty to others is unacceptable and can result in the loss of privileges, possessions, and, most important, your positive regard.

Tough Choices

One of the more difficult situations that parents confront is when they've made an honest effort to help their son live up to his potential within a particular school, only to discover that for whatever reason it seems unlikely to happen. Sometimes we wait too long to consider the possibility of transferring to another school or to arrange for an alternative education plan or do whatever else might be necessary for a boy to thrive. We should not be limited by our own experiences as children. There are many more schools available now, and parents have a multitude of choices about how to go about educating their children. Sometimes you can transfer to another school within your school district by paying an additional fee, or perhaps your child can attend a private school. Many districts have special academies within their regular schools, and charter schools abound. Even home schooling is a possibility sometimes, with a few caveats.

My personal perspective is that home schooling should be an option only when there are no others. While it sometimes meets the needs of individuals in special circumstances, most home-schooled children miss the opportunity for social interaction with peers *in a communal setting*, which is important to their life experience and emotional development. Other arrangements for social interaction, although helpful, cannot replicate the diversity of personalities, perspectives, and experiences that a child will encounter in school. (Unfortunately for some home-schooled children, this is precisely the point, as some parents wish to limit their exposure to ideas and ideals that diverge with their own. While this desire can stem from honorable intentions, it's a recipe for dependence or rebellion.) If mastery of information were the only purpose of education, we could close our schools. Instead, schools are cornerstones of our communities; they reflect and develop our goals, values, and leadership. As we've discussed, many boys have difficulty connecting with others, and it's important to provide them with as many opportunities as possible to meet new people and discover that they're not alone.

So when do you know if it's time to move on? The stress of changing schools is real; there is a risk of losing ground academically if curricula vary; there are often factors of transportation, cost, and even residence to consider. When you have multiple children, the situation can grow even more complicated. Yet if your son is unhappy, is

developing a dislike of school, or isn't able to achieve appropriate social and academic milestones, you can't afford to waste time—if
you've exhausted efforts to make his current school work. Seek advice from others you trust and let your instinct and judgment guide
you. Does your son want to switch schools? Sometimes children give
up on the notion of enjoying their education and resist switching
schools because they feel it's hopeless. Or they may balk at leaving
because in their minds a "known evil" is better than an unknown. Yet
as often, boys realize that they aren't doing well and are grateful
when you help them manage a transition. Be sure to take your son's
perspective into consideration.

The foundation of many of the interventions and ideas that we
discussed in this chapter is a thorough assessment. In the next chapter I'll give you some specific guidelines about when professional help
is required. We'll also talk about the components of a psychological,
or what is sometimes called a psychoeducational, evaluation and how
it might help your son.

ELEVEN

When Professional Help Makes Sense

■ ■ ■

By now you probably have an idea of whether you can manage any concerns you have about your son's communication abilities on your own. In Chapter 7, I offered some indications of when you might want to have your son tested for a neuropsychological problem. And all the boys whose stories you've read, along with the checklists in Chapter 1, should have given you a sense of where your son fits along the continuum of communication abilities and social competence. If you believe a professional evaluation of your son might be warranted, read on to learn about what kind of professional help is available and how to find the right person to assist your son. Even if you don't think you need this kind of help right now, you might find it helpful to read this chapter, because there may be a time in the future when collaboration with a professional will be in your son's best interest. If you have any doubts about whether to call in a professional, the following criteria should help you gain some perspective.

How Do You Know If Your Son Needs Professional Help?

Whether or not your son requires professional help is a somewhat subjective judgment that will likely be based on a number of factors. Most parents don't want to leap prematurely into getting a psychological evaluation, but they also don't want to waste time if professional help will make important differences in their son's life. So it's helpful to have some basic rules of thumb for deciding whether to work with someone outside your family to bring about change in your son's communication and social behavior.

The following are some solid indicators that suggest professional help may be warranted. Keep in mind that any conclusions you draw, and actions you choose to take, will likely be guided by your response to multiple questions or areas of concern.

■ *Your son's teacher has independently raised the same concerns about your son's social behavior as you have.* This gives you mounting evidence that his problem is pervasive. A teacher's perspective may be particularly valuable because teachers are accustomed to seeing children your son's age and have a good sense of what is "normal" for his peer group.

■ *You're beginning to see a self-esteem problem emerging as the result of social communication deficits or social awkwardness.* It is simply unacceptable to allow a boy's self-esteem to suffer as the result of untreated learning or social problems.

■ *You have no adequate explanation for your son's social behavior, or his behavior is puzzling or mysterious.* One of the key purposes of an evaluation is to provide an explanation, not just data (we'll talk more about this later).

■ *You're applying interventions consistently, but they are rarely effective.* A professional may be able to offer guidance in working with the subtleties of your son's behavioral challenges. If you discover that the things you try from self-help or parenting books take you only so far, it may be time to have a detailed assessment done. Understanding your son's actions and emotional needs will bring form to how you respond to him.

■ *Your son's social problems have gotten so severe that you're concerned about whether he can stay in his current school or you're confused about the value of a transfer or the best place to transfer to.* Children are often deeply affected by a change in their environment, even when they can't express those feelings. Before you make such a change, it might be beneficial to make sure you've explored all the options for making his current situation work, provided there's no immediate danger to his health or emotional welfare. Sometimes a specialist can give you some guidance about how to present such a change to your son in an encouraging, supportive way.

■ *You're having serious disagreements with your spouse or other care-givers about how to respond to your son's social challenges.* Boys consistently respond well to seeing solidarity between parents and among various support professionals. The more visible you make that solidarity, the easier it is for boys to accept your expectations and apply their energy toward meeting them. Therapy often provides the critical difference in smoothing out disagreements and helping a family adopt a team approach.

■ *Your son has been treated for a behavioral problem such as ADHD by your family doctor, and your family doctor now feels that his behavioral challenges have grown beyond the scope of his or her expertise.* A mental health professional can help you determine whether behavioral treatment would be a helpful addition to medication. Studies repeatedly indicate that integrating medication and behavioral psychotherapy is effective for a wide variety of behavioral and emotional problems in children. Ideally, your son should have a comprehensive evaluation before starting any medication, to rule out other potential causes of behavior problems and to support important decisions about medication.

■ *You notice that one of your son's skill areas is significantly below other areas of achievement.* For example, his reading comprehension is lagging behind his reading fluency skills; his math skills are lagging behind his reading; or he is fine academically but has some social learning deficits. Your son may have some type of specific learning anomaly. All of these problems warrant attention by a professional who can determine why that deficit may be present and what you can do about it.

■ *Your son is trying his very best but is still not succeeding.* Your son may have been put in a position of high stress and is probably feeling a great deal of discomfort with that pressure. Nothing can make a boy feel helpless faster than getting nowhere despite his best efforts.

Who Can Help?

When your son has a problem that seems to require professional intervention, many sources of guidance are available to you. The person or people required to help him will vary according to his individual challenges, your location, and your ability to access resources. Your first task is to know what your options are.

Psychologists

Psychologists generally hold a doctoral degree, typically a PhD, PsyD, or EdD. While they spend much of their time providing psychotherapy, many psychologists also complete detailed diagnostic evaluations, including specialized testing when needed. Although some psychologists identify themselves specifically as "child" practitioners, there are many others who treat people of various ages, including children and adolescents. Ask about a psychologist's training and clinical focus before undertaking evaluation or treatment. You will be looking for someone with experience in working with boys your son's age who understands both the psychology and neuropsychology of social development. This type of qualified professional is often an excellent starting point for investigating your son's needs. The field of psychology encompasses diverse kinds of knowledge, and most psychologists have working relationships with allied professionals. A competent practitioner will be able to do an evaluation that helps you understand the scope of your son's problem and the various types of intervention he might benefit from.

Psychiatrists

Psychiatrists, particularly those focusing on children's issues, are the best choice when your son needs medication to assist with behavioral or emotional regulation. Psychiatrists have medical degrees, can prescribe medication, and will monitor your son for side effects and drug interactions. Unfortunately, child psychiatrists are in short supply in many areas, making it necessary to consider other options for medical intervention. In some cases, family doctors or pediatricians will prescribe psychotropic (for the brain and mind) medications. Many psychologists enjoy collaborative and fruitful relationships with physicians in these specialties. (I've often found that family doctors and pediatricians are willing collaborators when it comes to consulting about the behavior or treatment of a child. The advantage of this type of communication and teamwork is nearly immeasurable when it comes to providing timely and responsive care!) However, some primary-care doctors prefer to refer children's behavioral health issues to a child psychiatrist. The decision to treat or refer often hinges on a doctor's familiarity with appropriate medications, the number of medications involved, and the severity of the problem to be treated. Don't be afraid to ask your doctor about her or his experience or to seek a second opinion if you have any questions about medication management. Finally, even if you're going to work with a psychiatrist, she or he is not likely to be trained in psychological testing or be able to commit the time necessary to complete the type of diagnostic evaluation your son may need. You'll still need a psychologist to clarify diagnostic concerns and track your son's progress through treatment.

Developmental Pediatricians

Developmental pediatricians are medical doctors who may be helpful when there seems to be a problem with some aspect of neurodevelopment such as a pervasive developmental disorder, learning disability, or ADHD. Physicians in this specialty quite often have significant expertise in the specifics of language development and a great appreciation for how language deficits interact with other cognitive functions. The expertise and guidance of these professionals can be very valuable, although in some areas of the country you may unfortunately have to wait months for an appointment. In my view, this is not acceptable when your son has emerging problems or you have pressing questions.

School Psychologists

School psychologists, who are often state certified rather than licensed, have been specially trained to address the academic and behavioral issues that affect children in school. Most school districts, if not each school, have access to the services of a school psychologist, who can help determine your son's intellectual ability and whether it is consistent with his achievement. Families often call school psychologists first when they have questions about the possibility of a learning disability in their son. These professionals are also on the front line of problem solving disruptive behavior in the classroom, including behavioral issues associated with ADHD.

Speech–Language Pathologists and Therapists

Speech–language pathologists are very helpful in identifying formal problems related to speech production or communication. Speech–language therapists are very familiar with the social communication challenges of children and can be especially helpful in supporting the development of pragmatic communication skills, a concern we've discussed throughout this book. If your son receives a school-based assessment for learning difficulties, referral to a speech–language therapist may be one important outcome of that evaluation. At the time of this writing, news reports were emerging about the nation's shortage of speech–language pathologists. Many of these professionals are recruited to higher-paying positions within hospitals and allied health care settings, making it increasingly difficult for schools to retain them. Competition for their services within schools can also be intense. Don't be surprised if you have to advocate strongly for such intervention within your son's own school. Sometimes a boy's difficulties with speech become apparent early in life, before he even starts school. At such times it's appropriate to contact a speech–language therapist directly so that your son gets the intervention he needs sooner rather than later—it will make a substantial difference in his social confidence.

Occupational Therapists

Occupational therapists are often helpful when boys are not demonstrating age-appropriate sensory processing or motor skills. These problems are often apparent when boys are still quite young. Helping boys gain better coordination and physical mastery, especially when they lag behind peers, is an important contribution to self-esteem and self-confidence. (Occupational therapy is clearly advised when there are genuine developmental issues. However, in some places, where there is immense pressure to gain acceptance to exclusive preschools, some parents have taken their toddlers in for occupational therapy to give their child an "edge" in motor skills. While intensive intervention might expedite the development of such skills, in my view this is potentially stressful and unnecessary for boys who would eventually achieve their motor potential on their own.)

Guidance Counselors and Other School Staff

Although we talked about the work of teachers in the preceding chapter, it's important to note the role of guidance counselors when your son is struggling with some aspect of social or emotional development. Guidance counselors are often responsible for devising specific programs and interventions in school and can provide a wealth of information about the resources a school district provides to help kids, both academically and socially. They can also provide on-site assistance for boys whose social developmental needs are most pressing within the school context, often working collaboratively with teachers and parents when problems occur in the classroom.

Your son's school may have other allied staff who take an active role in assisting with his development. Whether it is a coach, school librarian, classroom aide, upperclass mentor, or parent volunteer, there are likely to be people willing and able to support your son in important ways. Sometimes the difficulty lies with finding out what help is available. In general, there are more resources available now than when you or I went to school, although there are also more children who qualify for that help.

The "Point Person"

In many cases, boys will benefit from the orchestrated effort of multiple specialists. When this is the case, it is usually advantageous to identify one specific professional as the "point person" through whom ideas, plans, and communication will be filtered. This is easier said than done, but it's worth the effort so you have someone to coordinate efforts and interpret the findings and advice of the different specialists involved. Everyone tends to see a problem from his or her own professional perspective and describe it in terms used in his or her own field. One mother came to me lamenting, "Look at these reports—I had no idea he had so many problems," about her eight-year-old. A psychologist had noted that he had a problem with phonological processing, an audiologist had reported a central auditory processing disorder, and a teacher described a reading comprehension problem for the same child. Essentially, they were all looking at the same issue from slightly different angles. I asked the boy's mother to think of it this way: "You're driving along and you get a flat tire. Your son says, 'The car's stopped.' Your husband says, 'These tires were just inspected.' Your daughter says, 'We're going to be late.' Your only problem is that you've got a flat tire, but it's just been analyzed in three different ways."

This usually results when those evaluating your son don't communicate with each other. Naturally, these people tend to be busy, and it's often difficult for them to reach others who may be working with your son. Also, unless you advise them of the others providing care and authorize them to release information to each other, they

can't communicate. However, such coordination is absolutely necessary to taking a team approach. *Parents who help organize communication
among those treating their son are likely to see their interventions work more
effectively.* I have found that a good approach is to periodically schedule meetings, or at least a phone conference, including pertinent individuals involved in your son's care. Physicians and therapists who
schedule on the hour, and teachers who are running a classroom, often find it difficult to fit in lengthy conversations otherwise. When it
can be achieved, this type of meeting ensures an integrative approach
to understanding and helping your son and allows for the level of attention required to yield good results.

Choosing Someone to Work With

When you've decided that you need the help of a professional, the
next natural question to ask is: who? This is an important consideration, because there are many people who can help in different ways
but might not necessarily be the right source of help for your child.

The Right Specialty

The first thing you need to decide is which type of professional
to consult. If you decide that a psychologist is a good choice, you'll
still need to determine which type of psychologist is best. If your
son's communication challenges seem to be primarily emotional,
such as refusing to talk to you or feeling very shy around peers, he
will probably do well with a psychologist who specializes in helping
with family dynamics or social anxiety. However, if your son has a
history of learning problems or is hampered by serious ADHD, he
may need someone who can assess and explain how those challenges
are related to whatever communication difficulties he's having. As
with other professionals, a psychologist's degree does not tell you everything you'll want to know. Most psychologists will field brief telephone calls to explain their backgrounds and expertise.

The Right Practitioner

Once you've identified the type of professional to start with, you
need to figure out how to find the right individual practitioner. One

important source of guidance is simple word of mouth. Talk to parents of your son's classmates or school personnel. Word of mouth generally reflects positive opinions based on personal experience. The Yellow Pages may be an easy source to use, but the ads give you relatively little information about a person's background, personality, or clinical expertise. In my own practice, after a few years of trying to cram too much pertinent information into a Yellow Pages ad, I developed a more comprehensive website, like many other clinicians. Another note about the phone book: the size of an ad doesn't indicate quality of care or depth of experience. While good and successful practices often do have large ads, other excellent clinicians have such busy practices that they minimize their advertising exposure—they simply have too many clients as it is.

Another way to find a competent professional is through the websites and directories of professional associations. For example, your state learning disabilities association may have a register of psychologists who specialize in treating children. Hospitals and universities may also have referral sources. Insurance companies usually provide a list of psychologists who are on their panels; criteria for inclusion vary widely, but most major insurers have basic standards providers must meet. State licensure boards also maintain lists of licensed professionals.

One thing to be aware of is that there are both publicly funded and private mental health providers, along with nonprofit organizations and public–private partnerships. In every state, there is a patchwork of programs and resources to meet mental health needs, and your access to quality, affordable care often depends on where you live. An important distinction relates to the inpatient versus outpatient delivery of care. Unless you're in a crisis situation, an office visit versus a hospital admission is what you should be seeking, and any inquiries you make of clinicians or insurers should be regarding their *outpatient mental health care*.

The Importance of Therapeutic Fit

For many parents, the ultimate factor in deciding whether or not a professional is right for their child is their perception of *therapeutic fit* at the first meeting. Although it can seem time-consuming and expensive to go to more than one initial evaluation, it actually isn't when you consider the consequences of working with the wrong person. It's important to feel confident and comfortable with the person who is going to help your child. You should leave that first meeting feeling as though the evaluator understands the issues that you are presenting, has given you at least some feedback about what the likely cause of your son's problems are, and has shown you further indication that she or he has a specific plan for finding out whatever additional information is required. In addition, you should feel as though the evaluator is someone you can talk to and who is open to discussing your son's challenges from multiple perspectives. If you don't feel as though you've been understood or if you think there's a mismatch between your son and the evaluator, consider looking for another clinician. This is one reason it's important to take your son to the initial interview. His presence gives him the opportunity to get a sense of the evaluator and to decide for himself if he or she is someone he would feel comfortable working with.

Here are some factors to consider in finding a clinician for your child.

Does she or he:

- Have an appropriate degree from a recognized university?
- Have a current, state-approved license?
- Appear to have a well-established, professional workplace?
- Belong to professional networks (professional associations, chamber of commerce, insurance panels, university affiliation)?
- Have experience working with boys your son's age?
- Possess appropriate evaluation materials? (Some psychological tests cost thousands of dollars. A clinician who has invested in these materials and the training to administer them probably has a commitment to working with children.)
- Have good word-of-mouth referrals?
- Demonstrate a willingness to disclose information about his or her training, experience, and philosophy?
- Exhibit a willingness to work collaboratively with you and other specialists?
- Relate well to you and your child?

These factors should count more heavily than convenience or expense in choosing a clinician. While the reality is that barriers involving location, scheduling, and cost can sometimes be too difficult to overcome, I hope that you will use all the resources at hand to make helping your child your highest priority. Chances are, the long-term consequences of inaction will outweigh any immediate roadblocks.

What Is a Diagnostic Interview?

Let's suppose you've decided to have a psychologist evaluate your son for a social learning or communication problem. The first step will be for you and your son, as well as his other parent, if possible, to participate in a diagnostic interview. This is typically your initial meeting, when you and your son will be asked a number of questions about your current concerns, his developmental history, and whether or not there are particular problems at school or at home that need to be addressed. Your answers will help determine if he has followed a typical course of development and will put your son's behavioral issues in context. The more candid and accurate you can be, the better. This interview is where a diagnostic impression will begin to be formed, but most likely not where it will be concluded. This is because a diagnostic interview, although it may last one to two hours, is not enough to form a complete clinical picture of what is psychologically occurring for a child. (Please note that my position on this matter contradicts the policies and expectations of many insurance companies and managed care organizations. However, one of the key reasons for poor therapeutic outcome is a failure to take the time to understand a problem thoroughly.) Go to the diagnostic interview with any other evaluations your son has had, notes about your observations of his behavior, and any other pertinent details from his school that might help a clinician form the most complete picture possible of his strengths and difficulties.

A diagnostic interview is typically not the time to begin working on therapeutic issues. Although it's appropriate to bring up concerns—for example, about how family members interact at home—it's not reasonable to expect immediate intervention for such problems. At this point the most important thing that a psychologist can do for you is to get a conceptual grasp of what is occurring for your son so that an informed intervention plan can be organized and put in place. There's an important distinction to be made between a *diagnostic interview* and a *diagnostic evaluation*. When we talk about a diagnostic evaluation, we're talking about not only the initial interview, but also about subsequent meetings, which may include testing or other examinations required to accurately understand your son's difficulties. Diagnostic evaluation can be a lengthy process, often involving several hours of your son's time spent one-to-one with the clinical examiner. In my own practice, it's not unusual for a child to be seen by more than one clinician. From our perspective, this is an advantage since you're then gaining the benefit of insight from multiple people, each of whom undoubtedly will have a slightly different perspective of your son's psychology and the factors that shape his behavior. Again, the most important thing is that all those who interview your son communicate with each other so that a consensus of opinion can emerge.

Before the diagnostic interview, it will be helpful to spend some time talking with your son about what is likely to take place. Younger children may need some help understanding the difference between a medical doctor and a "talking doctor." Certainly, it's important to avoid threatening or disparaging talk such as "If you don't straighten out, I'm taking you to a shrink," or "Just wait until I tell the doctor what's been going on." More subtle negative messages, such as "If this behavior doesn't change, I'm afraid we'll have to see someone about it," can also reinforce feelings of guilt or anxiety. I would suggest being brief, low-key, and positive. If you spend a lot of time building up the pending appointment, your son is likely to suspect you of "overselling," and you also open the door for argument and refusal. Something along the lines of "We're going to see someone who has been helpful to boys who are having difficulties like you. We'll see how it goes" should be sufficient, unless he expresses a lot of concerns.

Older boys should be encouraged to ask questions during the interview and to express themselves freely. Many boys are averse to the diagnostic process, because it tends to put them in the spotlight, and having to articulate their responses to questions can be uncomfortable. (Remember, when boys are being evaluated for communication problems, we can expect them to have communication difficulty in a context like a diagnostic interview!) A skillful clinician can often mitigate this difficulty. It's important that you be supportive of the whole process and express optimism about the potential outcome. Your son should understand that you're taking him to the interview not to punish him or because you feel something is "wrong" with him, but because you want to be well informed and assist him to achieve his best. When you're very matter-of-fact, your son won't feel unnecessarily stigmatized by going to see a mental health professional.

Finally, after the diagnostic interview, talk with your son on the drive home. Please encourage him to tell you about his impression of the process and the therapist. This will help you know whether you've found a good therapeutic fit. I would advise you to listen carefully to your son and to trust his instincts. Boys will usually let you know when they feel connected, even though they may not spell that feeling out in so many words.

What If He Won't Participate?

At the same time, you'll need to use your parental instincts to differentiate between a poor fit and a boy who would be resistant to working with virtually anyone. When faced with the latter situation, consider calling the psychologist to discuss the situation and brainstorm ideas for building a better working alliance. This reinforces that you won't let your son's defiance discourage you, as well as the notion that problems are meant to be solved, not avoided. This is what happened when Jennifer, a busy single mother with an angry and reluctant fourteen-year-old son, called me. His problems were substantial enough that she considered therapy imperative. "I know he really needs some help, but he says he won't come to therapy." Jennifer and I considered a variety of possibilities, including having an uncle her son admired talk to him in different terms, about losing privileges, or offering incentives. When I finally met Jennifer's son, I asked her how she got him to the appointment. "I did everything," she laughed. "Well, I told him that I wasn't willing to drive him around anymore if this wasn't one of the stops. My brother came over and talked to him. He's a vet, a no-nonsense type of guy, and my son worships the ground he walks on. He told him that it was okay if he didn't want to go for long-term therapy, or if he wanted to switch therapists, but he expected him to give it an honest effort before deciding against it. He said, 'If you can look me in the eye and tell me you gave it your best shot but it wasn't helpful to you, then you'll hear no more about it from me. But I'll know if you're telling the truth.' The crème de la crème was when he said, super-casually, 'But if you get yourself straightened out, you might be old enough to come up with me to my hunting lodge for a week or so.' That did it."

Considering the nature of her son's problems and his resistance to any form of intervention, Jennifer applied appropriate pressure, with the resources she had, to get her son to try therapy. Later, her son thanked her. "If I had waited, I'd have probably gotten into some bad stuff," he said. If your son is refusing help he badly needs, your first consultation with a therapist may be to determine how to engage him in therapy. Some parents, especially those with older or angry sons, come to therapy without their sons at first. This gives them an opportunity to strategize about how to support positive change in the home to the point where their sons will be receptive to accepting their offers of help.

The Rest of the Diagnostic Evaluation: What Types of Testing Might Your Son Need?

A good evaluation requires not only competent administration of tests but also a high degree of reasoning to establish what issues are to be explored and which assessment tools will be most useful. Sometimes clinicians have to probe like detectives, administering tests either to rule out or zero in on suspected problems. This is why your evaluator may not be able to give you a comprehensive list of tests to be administered at your first meeting. Psychologists who administer "boilerplate" testing protocols may not be looking at your child with an ideal level of specificity, although in some cases, such as when the assessment is very narrow in scope, it may be sufficient. Beyond the science of administration, the art of interpretation is critical—an experienced clinician will make sense of the pages of data that an evaluation yields and be able to draw an accurate and insightful portrait of your son's state of mind. Following are some basic types of assessment your son might need, as well as some sample excerpts from psychological reports to illustrate the type of information you can gain from a good evaluation.

Intellectual

It's generally a good idea to have some type of intelligence testing done when any type of neuropsychological or cognitive evaluation is being undertaken. In addition to getting some baseline data about your son's intelligence, this type of testing will help you put your son's social behavior in context with respect to his cognitive abilities. This is because "IQ" tests are composed of a dozen or more subtests, which provide very specific information about your son's learning challenges and strengths. This may help explain specific learning deficits and assist with the selection of school curricula and will provide an overall good clinical picture of your son's neuropsychological functioning. Many of the evaluations conducted by my own practice begin with the administration of the Wechsler Intelligence Scale for Children (WISC), a "practice standard" when it comes to evaluating children's intelligence. I don't believe that the WISC is the first and last word on a child's intellectual ability, but the test does provide a wealth of information about where a child is likely to succeed more easily in school and where he might need special intervention. I also believe that, when interpreted correctly, the WISC can provide very good information about your son's social cognitive skills.

EXAMPLE

Overall, Dale's WISC profile suggests he does his best work when required to solve problems with unambiguous solutions. He is significantly more challenged by tasks that require subtle perception and interpretation of complex verbal concepts. He also struggles with executive control skills related to planning and organization. This seems to explain his difficulty organizing his desk at school and why he is often late with homework. Conversely, one of Dale's strengths is being able to sustain attention and work diligently at two- and three-dimensional problems. Dale is clearly more comfortable with nonverbal problem solving. Finally, although WISC data are typically very reliable indicators of cognitive ability, Dale's performance appeared to be affected by fatigue (occasional yawning). Retesting at some future time may reveal an IQ at least several points higher than the current results suggest. . . .

There are several other prominent intellectual tests as well, all of which provide information relatively similar to that provided by the WISC. Some parents hesitate to have their child's intelligence tested because they fear hearing that their son has average, or below average, intelligence. We all need to remember that intelligence tests, while valuable from a clinical perspective, particularly in terms of predicting academic performance, do not measure the multiple ways of knowing people possess. They do not measure a person's value, insight, or capacity for happiness and success. Each is but one tool from a box of many, and the results should be integrated with a judicious perspective. Of note is that the encouragement of the clinician, and the readiness of your son, along with other factors, can impact the scores. (A child who is sleep deprived, ill, or upset should have his testing rescheduled.) This is why such tests are sometimes administered more than once over the course of a child's schooling.

Achievement

Achievement tests are less focused on your son's ability than on his actual level of accomplishment, typically with respect to his academic skills. For many years most schools and government agencies have defined a learning disability as a statistical discrepancy between a child's *ability* and a child's *achievement*. Currently this model for determining a specific learning disability is changing, but the assessment of achievement is still valuable because it determines whether or not a child is performing at a level consistent with his capabilities. Some achievement test batteries can be broken down into very specific components. A personal favorite of mine is the Woodcock–Johnson Psychoeducational Battery, which, for example, when you want to evaluate math skills, examines up to four specific areas of math and quantitative analysis. Achievement tests can also help you understand your son's oral comprehension, reading comprehension, and written expression. All of these basic abilities are related to social communication.

EXAMPLE

Despite Bernard's strong performance on other Woodcock–Johnson tests, his difficulty synthesizing phonemes helps to explain his problems with reading fluency and confirms previous determination of a central auditory processing disorder. Still, the current evaluation finds that Bernard is able to discriminate target auditory input from background noise when performance anxiety is decreased. The possibility that social and emotional factors inherent in a classroom environment are affecting Bernard's auditory processing skills should be considered. Specifically, it is not uncommon for children to be more anxious in group situations where they have less control over the pace of interaction and level of reciprocal communication. . . .

Attention Deficits

ADHD has come a long way with respect to how it is understood and assessed. Current test protocols are more sophisticated and capable of helping examiners understand the nuances of how ADHD manifests in a particular individual. Often, when parents comb the Internet or collect information from books, they read or hear the statement "There is no test for ADHD." This is both true and deceptive. It's true that there is no test for ADHD in the sense that there is no blood test or brain scan, as there might be for some type of metabolic disorder or other form of physical pathology. Conversely, there are in fact psychological tests for ADHD that help an experienced evaluator place your son's attention, concentration, and impulse control within context.

Currently there are two basic varieties of ADHD tests. There are self-rating scales that are typically completed by parents and teachers (and often compared), which consider a boy's behavior within the normal flow of life. There are also what are called *continuous performance tests*. These are computer-based tests that require your son to respond to stimuli on a monitor, measuring his ability to both sustain attention and control impulsivity. I believe that an integration of both types of testing is extraordinarily useful.

EXAMPLE

Patrick completed computer-based neuropsychological testing for ADHD with medication (Concerta, 36 milligrams in the morning). Results suggest that his ability to sustain attention is normal with respect to his peer group. However, even with medication, Patrick demonstrated a significant problem with impulsivity. This finding was also reflected on rating scales completed by his teacher and teacher's aide, both of whom indicated that Patrick seems motivated to succeed and expresses a positive attitude, but has great difficulty remaining seated, waiting his turn, and speaking at appropriate times, particularly during interaction with peers. At the present time, Patrick's problems with impulsivity are undermining his potential to achieve academically at a level consistent with his ability. Patrick will be referred back to his pediatrician for reevaluation of medication options. . . .

In addition, since ADHD is really a reflection of a broader and more complex problem with executive awareness, it is often advantageous to administer psychological testing that examines different aspects of *executive control,* such as working memory, initiation, planning and organization, and self-monitoring, which we discussed in Chapter 7.

Social Cognitive Skills

Assessing social thinking skills is one area of evaluation that requires a high level of expertise in relatively subtle psychological functions. Often the assessment of social cognitive skills is done by "reading between the lines" in the data of other tests. Social thinking skills are concerned with how accurate a boy's social perception is and whether he can draw appropriate inferences from social observations. I prefer using a diverse constellation of tests, including those that require interpretation of facial expressions and body language, the construction of stories, comprehension of social situations, and the application of social language. These assessments are often found within test batteries designed for other purposes but are very useful when it comes to understanding social thinking skills. I particularly value using projective tests that require a child to construct stories from a series of picture cards with ambiguous meanings and content. I have repeatedly found that a child's ability to detect emotion in these cards, and how he constructs descriptions of what he sees, is a good measure of his capacity for more abstract emotional thought. Very concrete and simplistic responses often indicate that his social perception may be much the same.

EXAMPLE

Overall, Yuri's stories demonstrated limited narrative ability. His projections suggest a child who has some ability to solve problems but who is inclined to suppress observation of strong emotions. This suppression of emotion may reflect Yuri's self-consciousness about often feeling so angry (and being asked about these feelings by adults). The concrete quality of language used in Yuri's stories also reflects underdeveloped expressive language skills, highlighting probable social difficulties relating to others. Primary psychological themes that emerged in Yuri's stories included his need to categorize people as "good" or "bad." This type of psychological perspective, while partially expected given Yuri's age, is often associated with social and emotional inflexibility. Results suggest that Yuri would benefit from learning how to be more receptive and flexible when interacting with others. . . .

The clinicians in my practice purposely administer projective tests well into the evaluation process, when boys have developed a level of rapport and comfort with their examiner. The data derived from such a test may ultimately be a better reflection of what your son is capable of, in terms of communication, than what was observed, for example, during his initial interview.

Personality

When we talk about the assessment of a child's personality, we are really talking about his social and emotional adjustment and how it affects his interaction with others. There are a variety of measures, some of which are administered by a professional and others completed by parents or children and adolescents themselves. Typically, a psychologist will be interested in such factors as whether or not a child feels satisfied with his life, how he relates to his family, and how he sees himself in comparison with peers. This dimension of assessment focuses on self-concept and also examines basic elements of a child's mental status such as depression and anxiety. This type of information may be derived from the completion of self-report scales but may also result from very useful tests such as the Rorschach (the famous ink blot test) and related projective measures described earlier. Again, it is in the integration of personality test data that the most accurate picture of your son emerges. Administering multiple personality tests will provide the most comprehensive and meaningful picture of his psychosocial functioning. When parental input is required on a personality test, having *both* parents' responses gives the examiner a well-rounded perspective of a child's social and emotional adjustment.

EXAMPLE

Harwick's profile suggests a child who is likely to have an argumentative interpersonal style, consistent with parental report. Harwick is a strong-willed child who can become defiant when he feels stressed or "put on the spot." Although he shows relatively little outward emotion, test data suggest he worries excessively, contributing to his current pattern of social avoidance. While Harwick has had his share of personal success in sports and academics, he seems to harbor feelings of inadequacy that keep him from taking chances that could potentially improve his self-confidence. Harwick is likely to be perceived by peers as aloof even though he desires greater social attachment. His frequent trips to the school nurse for complaints such as fatigue, headaches, and stomachaches reflect his need for nurturing attention. Harwick will benefit from learning how to constructively seek that attention in a more direct manner. Intervention should be focused on helping him make a more accurate appraisal of his abilities, and supporting his need to take healthy social risks. . . .

And the Recommendations Are?

One of the primary things to keep in mind when considering the skill of an evaluator is that the benefit of an assessment is the degree to which the evaluator can interpret test results in a way that is meaningful to your son's treatment. This may sound like an obvious expectation, but it's often missing in an evaluation. Meaningful interpretation occurs when the evaluator understands the psychological and social dynamics of the challenges your son faces so that the information gathered can be applied in a relevant way. Currently in the field of psychology there is a strong movement toward empirically supported treatments and assessment procedures. While this is admirable in that it seeks to ensure quality and conformity with respect to the kinds of treatment that psychologists offer, equally important are the process of clinical judgment and the undeniable art of psychological assessment. If no art were involved in the process, it would simply be an algorithm that anyone could follow, and the results would all be interpreted in the same way. But, in fact, a good evaluation involves a high degree of interpretation and a sophisticated understanding and integration of the different levels of data derived from the assessment process. A good clinician will often put into words what you may have sensed and give you new insights into the way your son perceives himself and how he experiences his world, his personal strengths, and his challenges, as well as the interventions most likely to maximize his capabilities. A poorly conceived evaluation may provide you with lots of data but fail to report these findings to you in a relevant or meaningful way.

The whole point of getting an evaluation is to know what can be done to help your son. While it may be very interesting to learn a lot about how your child's mind works, ultimately as a parent you are most interested in what you can do to help. For this reason the recommendations section of an evaluation may be the part that you're most interested in. When meeting with someone to discuss the possibility of doing an evaluation, you may wish to ask about the extent of recommendations that will be offered at the conclusion of the evaluation. You may also wish to ask whether those recommendations will be very specific or of a more holistic nature, integrating various aspects of your son's social and emotional functioning. In whatever form recommendations are provided, they should not be generic, but instead should point to the specific strengths and challenges of your child. They should also address the specific concerns that brought you in for assessment and treatment. I hope that the recommendations will also point to how all those involved with your son can work in an orchestrated and coordinated manner to be of most help. When I see evaluations that suggest referral to other professionals, I'm usually encouraged that the evaluator has an open mind about who can be of assistance. The point of an evaluation is not to showcase the examiner's expertise but rather to pinpoint what is happening regarding your son and to talk about what can be done to help him.

It's Worth It

One of the primary barriers to getting children the evaluation they need is that for most people it's not only time-consuming but expensive. Psychological evaluations can cost up to several thousand dollars and may not be completed for weeks or even months, because multiple meetings between your child and a psychologist are often required. For younger children especially, sustaining the attention and energy necessary to perform up to their ability is very difficult in a day-long testing session. Consequently, test administration may be scheduled over multiple days or weeks, in one- to two-hour blocks. In addition, the psychologist will have to score and interpret all the tests and then write a report summarizing the findings. The work involved in integrating various types of data makes this an extraordinarily time-consuming task.

Although the time involved in doing an assessment is extensive, in my view it's also a great benefit. This is because time spent with your child is time spent getting to know him and how his mind works. Ultimately, this expedites treatment because it helps the psychologist develop a plan that will address his needs early on.

Another advantage of having a psychological evaluation done is that it establishes baseline data for your son, providing a point of comparison if he needs to be tested in the future. An assessment can be very helpful to schools by providing a roadmap for intervention that will help with a boy's academic performance and social interactions in the classroom. In addition, some parents find it valuable to have the evaluation of an independent examiner when they're at odds with a school's perspective of their son's needs. Knowing as much as possible about your son puts you in a stronger position to guide him. It will help you and your son make decisions that will draw on his natural strengths and help you creatively accommodate or improve areas of weakness. When you have a good understanding of your son's abilities and potential, you can encourage his involvement in activities where he's likely to experience success. You can use those successes to build his self-confidence and encourage him to expand his talents in areas, such as social communication, that may be more difficult for him.

When necessary, deciding to seek professional help expresses your care for your son and your commitment to meeting his developmental needs. Sandra, the mother of a six-year-old who was having behavioral problems, related it this way: "I had been hesitating to take Jay in to see someone, and it wasn't because I didn't want some help or an outside perspective; it was because I didn't want my mother to think I wasn't a capable parent. I imagined her saying, 'We never had to take you to a therapist!' But I realized that my job was not to impress her; it was to do the best I could for my son. The psychologist gave me some advice about communicating with my mother, who still thinks Jay's problems should be dealt with inside our family. But you know what? Even she has noticed a big difference in Jay. She feels like she can be closer to him."

■ ■ ■

Throughout the preceding pages we've touched on many ways that we can help and support our sons. People in the helping professions are available to you when it comes to making decisions that affect your son's future. Please accept the help and support of those you trust and cultivate a group of people you can turn to when you have questions or concerns. Far from reflecting any type of weakness, your ability to recognize when professional help is needed and your willingness to act on that intuition is a sign of your competence and strength as a parent. Involving a professional in your son's life does not replace you or diminish the value of your contribution to his development. It can, however, provide you with the understanding and tools needed to make important differences in his life.

Epilogue
The Men They Will Become

■ ■ ■

As adults we come to know that life is short, highlighted by experiences that underscore both its beauty and its temporality. Rather than sadden us, this knowledge intensifies our appreciation of life; what will be gone tomorrow can be cherished today, our sights set on the things that matter most, the things that hold their value across generations. Perhaps the most beautiful things in our world are evanescent or evolving. Childhood is one of these things, transforming a person before our eyes and reminding us that time is precious. As we reflect on how we can best support our sons on their trek to manhood, we can keep in mind that this beautiful time—when we are at the center of our sons' universe, at least for a while; when we have the awesome privilege and responsibility of raising them to be men—won't last.

"Before you know it, they're all grown up!"

"I'd give anything to have them be little again, just for a day."

These are the kinds of things we've all heard older parents say when they look back at how quickly time with their own children has passed. As parents, our busy lives can make it hard to catch our breath and appreciate the opportunity before us. Perhaps we sense that opportunity best when we peek in on our sleeping children after an exhausting day and pause in wonder. It's a scene often reenacted in literature and film, because it captures how awestruck we are at the miracle of our children's lives—at how children make us feel as if we've found life's meaning, our most important purpose. We translate that realization into the effort we put into raising our sons well, into finding an answer to the central question explored in this book: *How should we raise boys?*

Only by starting with this fundamental question can we challenge our assumptions and pause to consider our values, asking ourselves what lessons of our sons' boyhood will endure. How do we support their social and emotional development, build their character, their capacity to love and be loved? What can we give them that will last a lifetime and carry on through the generations? Perhaps our exploration has helped you discover perspectives or find answers that ring true for you and your family. If your son is having a problem, I hope you've found some assistance in the preceding pages. I especially hope you'll act on these realizations now, this very day, to make family life and your son's development all that it can be.

Years ago it was said that educating women would harm their ability to bear children; women were denied the vote on the grounds that they were incapable of logic. I'm sure that well-meaning parents of the day accepted these "truths" and encouraged their daughters toward fulfillment in the limited arenas available to them. Yet I'm just as sure that there were parents who not only loved but also *knew* their daughters. They did not allow the overwhelming consensus of society to blind their eyes to the fact that their daughters had far greater potential than was commonly assumed, and they fostered their daughters' intellectual development accordingly.

In a society in which women are denied education, the intellectual capital of half its members is underdeveloped. In our culture, the social and emotional development of men has been short-changed, and its negative impact has been felt across all levels of society, expressed in family discord, unemployment, men's health issues, violence, and crime. Social perspectives don't change quickly, but evolve from the open minds and courageous actions of a few. We cannot expect, or wish, to rewrite the scripts for masculinity overnight, but we can question whether we're limiting our sons by accepting outdated assumptions regarding their capabilities.

There is a societal expedient for men to evolve emotionally and communicatively. Right now the door is open for our sons to achieve new levels of social and emotional awareness and to avoid disenfranchisement and alienation. Those who "make the cut" will succeed, and those who follow old standards are in danger of being left behind. Remember that when we talk about change, it's always a matter of degree. Changing our vision of boyhood even modestly will yield major benefits for our sons. Just as losing 15 percent of your body weight or improving your golf score by 10 percent can have exponentially positive consequences, our sons' lives will feel extraordinarily different to them if their social communication skills are improved to an equivalent extent.

Make no mistake about it: the impetus for this social evolution flows not from political correctness but from sheer necessity. When we discuss the supports lacking for boys, it is not to compare their experience with girls' or to deny inequities on the other side of the gender aisle. It is not reasonable or even possible to reshape the behavior of a gender based only on ideology. Rethinking the nature of boys, and who we want them to become as men, must grow from our own emerging awareness of what it means to be a successful male. When we consider boyhood in this way, we're adopting a child-centered perspective of boys because we're focusing on what it feels like to *them* to grow up in our culture. If we are to maintain that child-centered perspective, we'll need to give due weight to how boyhood feels to boys.

In considering how social communication skills enhance and shape the identity of men, I've stressed the psychology of boys. When we grasp how boys think and feel, we are better positioned to make the pivotal choices that shape their social and emotional development. Remarkably, parents who take part in this process are bucking the tide of history. Who drew the line down the middle of the page and wrote "boys are" and "boys aren't" at the top of each column? Who decides what traits are on the list? Let's enjoy all the wonderful things that boys are and encourage a more integrated perspective that truly frees boys from age-old stereotypes. These male clichés limit the possibility of personal growth and encumber males to behave in ways that no longer meet the needs of a highly interconnected, global society.

What will the future hold for our sons? Will we continue to see vocations emerge that demand sophisticated interpersonal communication? Will the current epidemic of poor communication within the business community continue to escalate? How will technology affect the way information is shared? As you consider these questions, think about how you might raise your son. He will not only have to meet the demands of this society but will also influence its trajectory.

Will he become a leader? If so, he will need to be provided with leadership skills, and we have to reflect those skills in how we live as parents.

There is both a social and a biological imperative to the needed revolution in male communication. On a biological level, our society has seen men's health suffer as the result of stress and underdeveloped coping skills. We know, for example, that men who are divorced in middle age tend to have health that fails much more dramatically than do women. We also have seen that in childhood males are much more vulnerable to neurological syndromes such as ADHD, learning disabilities, and autism. Finally, in adulthood we've seen the enormous impact of stress on men's lives, and by extension, on the lives of their families. When we talk about building communication skills, we're also talking about building psychological resilience. It is through communication that we connect with other people, creating the relationships that are the very essence of resilience. If we love our sons, what could be more important than imparting to them the resilience necessary to live a long and healthy life? In this way, perhaps we can begin to redefine our notions of what strength means. Maybe we can expand our concept of strength to include a well-developed spirit fueled by a rich social and emotional life.

This social evolution must happen within a changing consciousness that is first rooted in family life. As I've tried to emphasize throughout this book, a heightened awareness of how our sons perceive other people and how their behavior causes them to be perceived by others is the beginning of this change in consciousness. Although there are many skills that we want to teach boys, teaching cannot begin until our own consciousness as parents has been transformed in such a way that we can appreciate who our sons are and who we want them to be. Sometimes this means breaking intergenerational cycles of dysfunction. When you look back and observe how masculinity has been expressed in your own family, have there been men who were socially and emotionally adrift? Often detached and ill equipped to cope with life's emotional changes, such men struggle to find meaning in their lives when the façades of work and status fall away. These are the consequences of a life focused on competition and accomplishment. Some may disagree with my thoughts, perceiving them as an attack on the virtues of accomplishment, but this is not the case. The drive for accomplishment is a dimension of maleness that needs redirection more than it needs change. We owe our sons the opportunity to consider complementary aspects of strength and masculinity. This is *accomplished* by shifting our own consciousness about what it means to be a boy or a man. And toward that realization we must verbalize and demonstrate that changing consciousness in our day-to-day lives.

Within recent years we have seen a significant change in patterns of college enrollment, with males occupying fewer and fewer slots in freshman classes. In part this reflects the growing aspirations of females, but it also seems to reflect a relative lack of preparation on the part of males for the demands of higher education. This gender schism is expected to increase substantially by 2010. One way that we will help our sons realize their potential is by giving them the confidence to succeed in social environments like school and work. Helping them feel comfortable in communities of communication, where knowledge is gained through attentive interaction with others, is one of our primary jobs as parents.

There are encouraging signs. Fathers seem to be more involved in raising their children almost everywhere we look. A few generations ago fathers were often relegated to the role of provider, family fix-it man, and occasional disciplinarian. The really great fathers were Little League coaches or scoutmasters. While these are still important and valuable roles, we now see dads becoming more involved and integrated in all aspects of family life. Listening to fathers, I hear their concern, reflected in good questions. They wonder about the reality of the neurological and behavioral syndromes that boys face. They ask direct questions about what they can do and what their role can be. These are very hopeful indications, and with encouragement men will pass on this level of inquiry and support to their sons.

Still, our society faces substantial challenges. These include the continued projection of stereotypes, school bullying, escalating stress, and the neurodevelopmental issues addressed by this book. Almost certainly, these issues will not disappear in our lifetime. The question we must ask ourselves is how much of a difference we can make. For example, if a school can reduce bullying by an observable margin, or if as a society we can downsize the number of prescriptions needed for attention and behavioral problems or decrease the rate of suicide among teenage boys, we're on the road to success.

Of course, these battles will not be won by improving social communication alone. Yet communication is the conduit that connects us to one another and also is how we are connected to our deeper selves.

We've talked about ways to build boys' self-awareness, even when this means asking them to remove the masks that both protect and obscure them. If we are to ask boys to be vulnerable, we must find and accept vulnerability within ourselves. If we are to ask boys to reach out, we must reach out to them. We cannot pull boys across the communication divide with our arms crossed in judgment or detachment, and they may not come of their own volition. The miracle of boyhood is that it's full of possibility, and the tragedy of boyhood is that it's over before you know what happened. Our job as parents is to turn boys' minds toward possibility, the moments of realization that instill hope, and give them the character they need to withstand the "slings and arrows" of the challenges to come. Hold your son. Talk with him. Make him laugh. Tell him what's in your heart and mind and free him to discover what's in his. By making boys more aware of their possibilities, we increase the likelihood that their potential will be fulfilled. In this century we will see people rise to accomplish things we can't now imagine. Yet whatever those accomplishments may be, if leaders are to lead, they will need to be able to relate to other people. Communication skills will not be optional when it comes to determining success in the twenty-first century.

Raising emotionally healthy boys is not a task for the timid or weak of spirit. It is a job for visionaries, parents who can see the men their sons will become. Parenting our children requires all the energy we can summon. It requires us to keep our wits, look with insight, and forgive ourselves when we make mistakes. It is both a job and a passion. And nothing we will ever do will be as important.

Helpful Resources

■ ■ ■

The following websites and books may be helpful in understanding and parenting boys with social communication challenges. Many of the ideas and strategies discussed in these resources are complementary to one another, assisting you to integrate multiple perspectives in helping your son.

Websites

Adam J. Cox, PhD
www.dradamcox.com
My website explores many of the topics discussed in this book, including information on parenting, social skills, and emotional literacy. I have also developed a free online newsletter for parents and teachers to comment on new developments in psychology and neuroscience relevant to the social development of children and adolescents. You will find a descriptions of workshop topics and information about how to schedule a presentation for your own school or organization. I look forward to meeting with parents and teachers and helping to implement communication and social skills training programs wherever they might be useful.

Anger

Center for Collaborative Problem Solving
313 Washington Street, Suite 402
Newton Corner, MA 02458-1626
Phone: 617-965-3000
www.explosivechild.com
Dedicated to understanding and meeting the behavioral challenges of

angry, inflexible children. Includes an innovative, well-defined approach to intervention amenable to the needs of most families.

Asperger Syndrome

Asperger's Connection
The Shriver Center
200 Trapelo Road
Waltham, MA 02452
Phone: 781-642-0229
www.ddleadership.org/aspergers

Interactive website that allows individuals with Asperger syndrome, their families, and anyone with an interest in Asperger syndrome to interact and support one another. Expert panels provide professional guidance and short courses to site visitors.

Autism Research Centre (ARC)
University of Cambridge
Douglas House
18b Trumpington Road
Cambridge CB2 2AH, England
Phone: 01223-746057
www.autismresearchcentre.com

Research program in the United Kingdom directed by Simon Baron-Cohen, PhD. Includes several tests that can be downloaded to assist in diagnosis of autism or Asperger syndrome.

Attention-Deficit/Hyperactivity Disorder

Children and Adults with Attention Deficit Disorder (CHADD)
8181 Professional Place, Suite 150
Landover, MD 20785
Phone: 800-233-4050
www.chadd.org

Comprehensive information about ADHD, including evidence-based treatments, new research, and links to individual state chapters of CHADD.

Early Childhood Development

Early Childhood Australia
P.O. Box 7105
Watson ACT 2602, Australia
Phone: 800-356-900
www.earlychildhood.org.au

Australian membership organization dedicated to advocacy for early childhood development. Relevant information for parents and teachers, as well as links to many other useful resources in Australia.

The Incredible Years
1411 8th Avenue W
Seattle, WA 98119
Phone: 888-506-3562
www.incredibleyears.com

Information on managing aggression and conduct problems in young children. Links to many resources for specific behavioral challenges, emphasizing research-based practices.

Emotional Literacy

Children's Social Behaviour Project
www.sussex.ac.uk/Users/robinb/csb

Longitudinal research program in the United Kingdom examining the social development and peer relations of elementary school children. Emphasizes implementation of strategies to assist socially isolated children in schools.

Childswork/Childsplay
P.O. Box 760
Plainview, NY 11803-0760
Phone: 800-962-1141
childswork.com

Distributes a wide range of therapeutic games, including those designed to improve social understanding, self-awareness, and prosocial behavior.

Collaborative for Academic, Social and Emotional Learning (CASEL)
Department of Psychology (M/C 285)
University of Illinois at Chicago
1007 West Harrison Street
Chicago, IL 60607-7137
Phone: 312-413-1008
www.casel.org

Promotes coordinated, evidence-based social, emotional, and academic learning as an essential part of education from preschool though high school.

Kids EQ: The Children's Emotional Literacy Project
www.kidseq.com

Advocacy organization dedicated to improving emotional literacy among children. Links to relevant books and resources.

Roots of Empathy
215 Spadina Avenue, Suite 160
Toronto, Ontario M5T 2C7, Canada
Phone: 416-944-3001
www.rootsofempathy.org
    Classroom-based parenting program in Canada that aims to reduce aggression through the fostering of empathy and emotional literacy. The program reaches children ages three to fourteen years.

Smallwood Publishing
The Old Bakery
Charlton House
Dour Street
Dover, Kent CT16 1ED, England
Phone: 01304-226800
www.smallwood.co.uk
    U.K. publisher of games and activities to facilitate social and emotional development. Appropriate for either school or home use.

Learning Disabilities

All Kinds of Minds
www.allkindsofminds.org
    Institute directed by Dr. Mel Levine, providing an integrative overview of learning disabilities, training for professionals, and Dr. Levine's approach to assessment.

Learning Disabilities Association of America (LDA)
4156 Library Road
Pittsburgh, PA 15234
Phone 412-341-1515
www.ldanatl.org
    National advocacy organization dedicated to disseminating information on learning disabilities and related legislation. Helpful in understanding your child's rights in school. Also includes links to LDA state chapters.

Learning Disabilities Association of Canada (LDAC)
323 Chapel Street
Ottawa, Ontario K1N 7Z2, Canada
Phone: 613-238-5721
www.ldac-taac.ca
    Useful information about learning disabilities and related resources in

Canada. Discuses school policies and legislation specific to Canadian education.

LDOnline
www.ldonline.org
Broad range of information about learning disabilities and their implications for academic and social development.

Schwab Foundation for Learning
1650 South Amphlett Road, Suite 300
San Mateo, CA 94402
Phone 800-230-0988
www.schwablearning.org
Membership organization that provides thorough discussion of learning disabilities, accompanied by lots of information on how families can effectively intervene to help children. Includes overview of auditory processing deficits and their relationship with learning challenges.

Specific Learning Disabilities Federation (SPELD) New Zealand
c/o Secretary
P.O. Box 25
Dargaville, New Zealand
Phone: 09-439-5955
www.speld.org.nz
Advocacy organization in New Zealand, providing information on learning disabilities, assessment and testing services, and assistance in working with schools.

Nonverbal Learning Disabilities

NLD on the Web
www.nldontheweb.org
Focuses on nonverbal learning disabilities and includes information on subtypes, diagnostic criteria, and links to parent-friendly resources.

Nonverbal Learning Disorders Association
2446 Albany Avenue
West Hartford, CT 06117
Phone: 860-570-0217
www.nlda.org
Useful information about nonverbal learning disorders and how they may be manifest at home and school. Includes suggestions for treatment options.

Parenting Advice/Discussion

Health Insite
Online Communications Section
Department of Health and Ageing, MDP 62
G.P.O. Box 9848
Canberra ACT 2601, Australia
Phone: 02 6289-8488
www.healthinsite.gov.au

Australian government organization providing comprehensive health information, including guidance for behavioral challenges among children. Includes many links to other Australian resources.

Kidsource Online
www.kidsource.com

Provides online forums for discussing parenting strategies for a variety of behavioral concerns related to children of all ages.

Natural Family Online
www.naturalfamilyonline.com

Addresses many common childhood developmental concerns. Emphasizes ideas and suggestions for a holistic approach to children's health, including behavioral difficulties.

New Horizons for Learning
P.O. Box 31876
Seattle WA 98103
www.newhorizons.org

Information for families with children who have special needs, including those who are gifted. Updates on neuroscientific research that may be helpful in determining your child's needs.

Parents Inc. (New Zealand)
P.O. Box 37-708
Parnell, Auckland, New Zealand
Phone: (64 9) 524 0025
www.parenting.org.nz

Community organization in New Zealand. Provides practical parenting guidance for a variety of behavioral issues, emphasizing the transgenerational impact of parenting.

Programs for Schools

Child Development Project (CDP)
Developmental Studies Center
2000 Embarcadero, Suite 305
Oakland, CA 94606-5300
Phone: 510-533-0213
www.devstu.org/cdp

Multiyear school program to improve learning skills and respectful connections among students, educators, and parents. Emphasizes integration of academic, social, and emotional goals and can be implemented at any school.

Psychologists

American Board of Professional Psychology
300 Drayton Street, Third Floor
Savannah, GA 31401
Phone: 800-255-7792
www.abpp.org

Contact information for board-certified psychologists in diverse clinical specialties, organized by state.

American Psychological Association
750 First Street, NE
Washington, DC 20002
Phone: 800-374-2721
www.apa.org

Largest professional organization of psychologists, providing a wide range of information to professionals and the public. Includes recommended resources for specific behavioral problems and information about how to find a qualified psychologist.

Social Anxiety

Social Phobia/Social Anxiety Association
2058 Topeka Drive
Phoenix, AZ 85024
www.socialphobia.org

Information about social anxiety and phobias, including diagnostic criteria, treatment options, and a moderated discussion of anxiety-related topics.

Speech, Language, and Communication

American Speech–Language–Hearing Association (ASHA)
10801 Rockville Pike
Rockville, MD 20852
Phone: 800-638-8255
www.asha.org

Extensive information on speech and language disorders, referral service to speech–language pathologists, and guidance about how they can potentially help your child.

National Institute on Deafness and Other Communication Disorders
National Institutes of Health
31 Center Drive, MSC 2320
Bethesda, MD 20892-2320
Phone: 301-496-7243
www.nidcd.nih.gov

Government site providing statistics on communication disorders, current programs of research, clinical trials, and training opportunities.

Books

Anger and Inflexibility

Greene, Ross W. *The Explosive Child*, HarperCollins, New York, 2001.
Greene, Ross W., & Ablon, J. Stuart. *Treating Explosive Kids: The Collaborative Problem-Solving Approach*, Guilford Press, New York, 2005.

Boys: More about Their Psychology and Behavior

Gurian, Michael. *Boys and Girls Learn Differently!*, Jossey-Bass, San Francisco, 2001.
Kindlon, Dan, & Thompson, Michael. *Raising Cain: Protecting the Emotional Life of Boys*, Ballantine, New York, 1999.
Macmillan, Bonnie. *Why Boys Are Different and How to Bring Out the Best in Them*, Barron's, New York, 2004.
Pollack, William. *Real Boys: Rescuing Our Sons from the Myths of Boyhood*, Holt, New York, 1998.

Brain-Based Gender Differences

Baron-Cohen, Simon. *The Essential Difference: The Truth about the Male and Female Brain*, Basic Books, New York, 2003.

Moir, Ann, & Jessel, David. *Brain Sex: The Real Difference between Men and Women*, Delta, New York, 1992.

Emotional Literacy

Goleman, Daniel. *Emotional Intelligence: Why It Can Matter More Than IQ*, Bantam, New York, 1997.
Gottman, John. *The Heart of Parenting: Raising an Emotionally Intelligent Child*, Simon & Schuster, New York, 1997.

Learning and Attention Problems

Barkley, Russell A. *Taking Charge of ADHD: The Complete, Authoritative Guide for Parents (Revised Edition)*, Guilford Press, New York, 2000.
Levine, Mel. *A Mind at a Time*, Simon & Schuster, New York, 2002.
Rourke, Byron P. *Nonverbal Learning Disabilities: The Syndrome and the Model*, Guilford Press, New York, 1989.
Thompson, Sue. *Nonverbal Learning Disabilities at School: Educating Students with NLD, Asperger's Syndrome and Related Conditions*, Routledge, London, 2002.

Medication Questions

Wilens, Timothy. *Straight Talk about Psychiatric Medications for Kids (Revised Edition)*, Guilford Press, New York, 2004.

Neurodevelopmental Issues

Gopnik, Alison, Meltzoff, Andrew N., & Kuhl, Patricia K. *The Scientist in the Crib: Minds, Brains, and How Children Learn*, Morrow, New York, 1999.
Healy, Jane M. *Endangered Minds: Why Our Children Don't Think*, Simon & Schuster, New York, 1990.

Social Skills

Nowicki, Stephen, & Duke, Marshall, P. *Helping the Child Who Doesn't Fit In*, Peachtree, Atlanta, 1992.

Bibliography

■ ■ ■

Barkley, R. A. (2006). *Attention-Deficit Hyperactivity Disorder: A Handbook for Diagnosis and Treatment, 3rd Edition*. Guilford Press, New York.

Baron-Cohen, S. (2003). *The Essential Difference: The Truth about the Male and Female Brain*. Basic Books, New York.

Berry, W. (1983). *A Place on Earth*. Farrar, Straus & Giroux, New York.

Blake, K. T., & Anderson, W. (2001). Social ability in children with dyslexia: "Refrigerator friendly" treatment suggestions. *International Dyslexia Association, Proceedings of 52nd Annual Conference*, Albuquerque, NM.

Bloom, L. (1993). *The Transition from Infancy to Language: Acquiring the Power of Expression*. Cambridge University Press, New York.

Bohart, A. C., & Greenberg, L. S., Eds. (1997). *Empathy Reconsidered: New Directions in Psychotherapy*. American Psychological Association, Washington, DC.

Bohnert, A. M., Crnic, K. A., & Lim, K. G. (2003). Emotional competence and aggressive behavior in school-age children. *Journal of Abnormal Child Psychology, 31*(1), 79–91.

Bruner, J. (1990). *Acts of Meaning*. Harvard University Press, Cambridge, MA.

Clark, C., Prior, M., & Kinsella, G. (2002). The relationship between executive function abilities, adaptive behaviour, and academic achievement in children with externalising behaviour problems. *Journal of Child Psychology and Psychiatry, 43*(6) 785–796.

Cohen, N. J. (2001). *Language Impairment and Psychopathology in Infants, Children, and Adolescents*. Sage, Thousand Oaks, CA.

Conlin, M. (2003, May 26). The new gender gap: From kindergarten to grad school, boys are becoming the second sex. *Business Week*, pp. 74–81.

Gardner, R. (2004, April 19). Under pressure. *New York*, pp. 34–39, 108.

317

Geschwind, N., & Galaburda, A. M., Eds. (1984). *Cerebral Dominance: The Biological Foundations.* Harvard University Press, Cambridge, MA.

Goleman, D. (1997). *Emotional Intelligence: Why It Can Matter More Than IQ.* Bantam, New York.

Gopnik, A., Meltzoff, A. N., & Kuhl, P. K. (1999). *The Scientist in the Crib: What Early Learning Tells Us about the Mind.* Morrow, New York.

Greenspan, S. I., & Benderly, B. L. (1996). *The Growth of the Mind and the Endangered Origins of Intelligence.* Perseus Books, Cambridge, MA.

Hart, B., & Risley, T. R. (1999). *The Social World of Children Learning to Talk.* Brookes, Baltimore, MD.

Healy, J. M. (1990). *Endangered Minds: Why Our Children Don't Think.* Simon & Schuster, New York.

Kimura, D. (2000). *Sex and Cognition.* MIT Press, Cambridge, MA.

Landy, S. (2002). *Pathways to Competence: Encouraging Healthy Social and Emotional Development in Young Children.* Brookes, Baltimore, MD.

Levine, M. A. (2002). *A Mind at a Time.* Simon & Schuster, New York.

Loney, B. R., Frick, P. J., Clements, C., Ellis, M., & Kerlin, K. (2003). Callous-unemotional traits, impulsivity, and emotional processing in adolescents with antisocial behavior problems. *Journal of Clinical Child and Adolescent Psychology, 32,* 66–80.

Macmillan, B. (2004). *Why Boys Are Different and How to Bring Out the Best in Them.* Barron's, New York.

Meunier, L. (1996, June 23). Gender and language use. Online contribution to *Gender and Postmodern Communication,* www.awn.mtansw.com.au/relevant_articles.htm.

Moir, A., & Jessel, D. (1992). *Brain Sex: The Real Difference between Men and Women.* Delta, New York.

Most, T., Al-Yagon, M., Tur-Kaspa, H., & Margalit, M. (2000). Phonological awareness, peer nominations, and social competence among preschool children at risk for developing learning disabilities. *International Journal of Disability, Development and Education, 47*(1), 89–105.

Nowicki, E. A. (2003). A meta-analysis of the social competence of children with learning disabilities compared to classmates of low and average to high achievement. *Learning Disability Quarterly, 26,* 171–188.

Nowicki, S., & Duke, M. P. (1992). *Helping the Child Who Doesn't Fit In.* Peachtree, Atlanta.

Ortiz, J., & Raine, A. (2004). Heart rate level and antisocial behavior in children and adolescents: A meta-analysis. *Journal of the American Academy of Child and Adolescent Psychiatry, 43*(2), 154–162.

Peterson, D. R. (2004). Science, scientism, and professional responsibility. *Clinical Psychology: Science and Practice, 11*(2), 196–210.

Real, T. (1997). *I Don't Want to Talk about It: Overcoming the Secret Legacy of Male Depression.* Scribner's, New York.

Restak, R. (2001). *The Secret Life of the Brain*. Dana Press and Joseph Henry Press, Washington, DC.

Rodkin, P., Farmer, T. W., Pearl, P., & Van Acker, R. (2000). Heterogeneity of popular boys: Antisocial and prosocial configurations. *Developmental Psychology, 36*(1), 14–24.

Rogers, C. R. (1961). *On Becoming a Person*. Houghton Mifflin, Boston.

Rosenthal, R. (1985). From unconscious experimenter bias to teacher expectancy effects. In J. B. Dusek, V. C. Hall, & W. J. Meyer, Eds., *Teacher Expectancies*. Erlbaum, Hillsdale, NJ.

Rossi, E. L. (1987). *The Psychobiology of Mind–Body Healing*. Norton, New York.

Salovey, P., & Sluyter, D. J., Eds. (1997). *Emotional Development and Emotional Intelligence*. Basic Books, New York.

Seligman, M. P. (1991). *Learned Optimism: How to Change Your Mind and Your Life*. Knopf, New York.

Shaywitz, S. (2003). *Overcoming Dyslexia: A New and Complete Science-Based Program for Reading Problems at Any Level*. Knopf, New York.

Sypher, H. E., & Applegate, J. L., Eds. (1984). *Communication by Children and Adults*. Sage, Thousand Oaks, CA.

Vygotsky, L. S. (1962). *Thought and Language*. MIT Press, Cambridge, MA.

Zigler, E. F., Singer, D. G., & Bishop-Josef, S. J., Eds. (2004). *Children's Play: The Roots of Reading*. Zero to Three Press, Washington, DC.

Index

■ ■ ■

Process-oriented speech, 97–98
Processing, language. *See* Language
Professional help
  deciding who to work with, 289
  for depression, 74
  determining need for, 279–281
  dialoguing with professionals,
    207–208
  options in, 281–286
  recommendations and, 298–299
Pronunciation, problems with, 176–
  177
Psychiatrists, 282–283
Psychologists, 282
Psychology, 17–25, 282
Public settings, verbalization and,
  48–49, 130–131
Public speaking, 130–131
Punishment, 174, 261–262

Q

Questions
  as answers to questions, 53
  of authority, 139–142
  detachment from, 111
  difficulty in answering, 47
  to elicit communication, 124
  length of responses, 99–100
  overquestioning by parent, 64,
    68–69

R

Raine, Adrian, 157–158
Randy's story (parental
  expectations), 202–203
Reading, 20, 168–170, 231–232,
  234
Reinforcement, 151, 155, 239
Rejection, fear of, 107
Relationships, 242–244
Religious community, 216

Resistance, 152–153
Resolution to problems, 65
Responses, 87, 99–100
Responsibility, 230
Rewards, 151, 155, 239, 261–262
Riley's story (anxiety), 100
Risk-taking, appropriate, 248–250
Rodney's story (emotional literacy),
  102
Role models, 64, 68
Royce's (learning disabilities), 166–
  167
Rules of communication. *See*
  Pragmatic communication
Russell's story (disruptive
  behavior), 262–263
Ryan's story (emotional awareness),
  66

S

Sarcasm, 64
Sassiness, 141
Scheduling, 197–201
Schemas for social communication,
  92–93
School
  alternatives to public schools,
    277–278
  attention during, 41
  bullying and, 273–276
  challenges for shy boys, 122–128
  changes in, 62
  changing, 280
  class size, 255
  co-ed/single-sex, 263–264
  competition and, 254
  counselors, 284–285
  difficult transition of, 126
  Does He Lack the Communication
    Skills Needed to Succeed
    Socially and Academically in
    School?, 32

About the Author

■ ■ ■

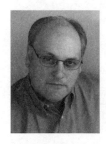

Adam J. Cox, PhD, ABBP, is a licensed and board certified clinical psychologist. He earned his doctoral degree in psychology at Lehigh University, Bethlehem, Pennsylvania, and completed his clinical training at Friends Hospital in Philadelphia. Dr. Cox became a psychologist from a nontraditional path. While working as a fine artist near New York City, he opened a studio and welcomed children who wanted to learn how to draw and paint. Getting to know these budding artists better, he discovered his passion for mentoring children, and has made that calling the focus of his career. He is the clinical director of Lehigh Psychological Services, a private group mental health practice in Emmaus, Pennsylvania, focusing on family and pediatric intervention. As an advocate for children's mental health, Dr. Cox is a frequent lecturer at national and international conferences. He has been quoted in a variety of national print media about a range of psychological issues affecting families and youth. These publications include *The New York Times, The Philadelphia Inquirer, Time, Family Circle*, and many others. Recently, he has made television and radio appearances in the Philadelphia area and has been featured on National Public Radio's *Voices in the Family*.